can health and nutrition interventions make a difference?

Davidson R. Gwatkin
Janet R. Wilcox
Joe D. Wray

with a foreword by Halfdan Mahler

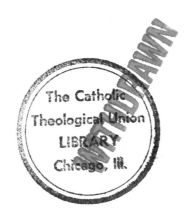

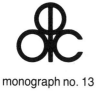

monograph no. 13

february 1980

The views expressed in this monograph are those of the authors and do not necessarily reflect those of the Overseas Development Council, its directors, officers, or staff.

Contents

Appendixes

Preface

Is our experience to date with health and nutrition interventions encouraging enough to justify augmented efforts to make primary nutrition and health care available to all? If so, what can we learn from our experience about how best to make primary care more widely available?

These are the issues we seek to explore. In doing so, we hope we can provide information of relevance to those who must decide how much emphasis is to be given to what kinds of intervention efforts. In particular, we hope that what follows can help identify strategies for the effective implementation of efforts of the kind proposed in the September 1978 Alma-Ata Conference on Primary Health Care—that it can help indicate an appropriate place for nutrition supplementation and education programs within broader primary care efforts, as well as within more general nutrition approaches that feature consumer-oriented production and distribution strategies. Above all, of course, we hope that our work will contribute to the fulfillment of the objectives of the International Year of the Child, in the context of which it was written: that it will help to improve the condition of the millions of unfortunate children around the world who, through no fault of their own, are destined to live so miserably and so briefly.

To the extent that our hopes are realized, the credit will be due in large part to the many who have so effectively encouraged and supported us. Our special thanks go to the United Nations Fund for Population Activities and the World Bank for their support. The UNFPA has been the principal source of financial assistance for the Overseas Development Council's work with child-oriented population strategies, of which this ODC/Harvard School of Public Health review of pilot project experience is an element. Such a detailed piece of work, however, would never have been undertaken or appeared in print had the World Bank not asked the ODC to contribute to its research report on "Nutrition, Basic Needs, and Growth"; and had the Bank not kindly granted ODC permission to prepare and publish this extensively revised version of what was originally a report to it. We also owe special debts of gratitude to many individuals: Alan Berg of the World Bank and our other fellow participants in the Bank's nutrition and basic needs study; the many field investigators who so graciously provided so much information about their projects and so many useful reactions to our earlier drafts; the organizers of the April 1979 Bellagio Meeting on Health and Population in Developing Countries—sponsored by the Ford Foundation, the International Development Research Centre, and the Rockefeller Foundation—for which an abridged version of this report served as a background paper; James P. Grant of the Overseas Development Council (soon of UNICEF); and Halfdan Mahler of the World Health Organization, who was kind enough to contribute the Foreword. None of the above, of course, is to be blamed for the many imperfections that remain.

Davidson R. Gwatkin
Janet R. Wilcox
December 1979
Joe D. Wray

Foreword

Halfdan Mahler
Director-General, World Health Organization

Nearly a billion people throughout the world are trapped in a vicious circle of poverty, malnutrition, and disease that saps their energy and greatly reduces their work capacity and impedes social development. Finding ways of breaking this circle so that these people can extricate themselves from their plight is one of the greatest social challenges that has ever faced humanity.

Many large-scale development schemes have been launched over the past two decades in response to this situation, but on the whole they have not lived up to expectations—despite large financial investments in their implementation. Often they have even been counterproductive. This has been as true of investments in the health sector as in any other sector. The failures have all had one thing in common: neglect of the all-important human factor. Economic growth had become an end in itself instead of being merely one of the means for ensuring genuine human development in social as well as economic terms. People were merely the incidental objects of development schemes. For example, in the health sector, all too often hospitals were constructed that were completely unmanageable from both the financial and the human viewpoints, but nevertheless were allowed to consume most of the limited health budgets available. Bricks and mortar and professional prestige were more important than the people to be served, and in any event these institutions could only provide services to a small elite in urban centers.

At the same time, donor agencies were becoming unduly complacent about the charity they were providing to the developing countries—measuring their assistance in terms of the money expended rather than in terms of the effect of that money on improving the lot of the people they were claiming to assist.

In recent years, a new understanding of development has begun to gain ground, giving rise to a completely different approach to international support for developing countries based on cooperation rather than assistance. In the health sector, the change in approach has been nothing short of dramatic. In May 1977, the Health Assembly of the World Health Organization decided that the main social target of governments and of WHO in coming decades should be the attainment by *all* the citizens of the world by the year 2000 of a level of health that will permit them to lead socially and economically productive lives. In 1978, the International Conference on Primary Health Care, held in Alma-Ata in the U.S.S.R., adopted a major declaration stating that primary health care is the key to attaining the target of health for all by the year 2000. The Alma-Ata Declaration described primary health care as essential health care based on practical, scientifically sound, and socially acceptable methods and technology made universally accessible to individuals and families in the community through their full participation and at a cost that the community and country could afford to maintain—regardless of their particular stage of development—in the spirit of self-reliance and self-determination. The Declaration called on all governments to formulate national policies, strategies, and plans of action to launch and sustain primary health care as part of a comprehensive national health system and in coordination with other sectors. It also called for urgent and effective international action—in addition to national action—to develop and implement primary health care throughout the world, and particularly in developing countries. In May 1979, the Health Assembly of the World Health Organization endorsed the Alma-Ata Declaration and invited member states to proceed with the formulation of strategies to attain the target of health for all.

The main pillars of these strategies are: 1) the political commitment of the governments and people of the world to introduce the necessary health reforms, 2) a multisectoral approach to health development as part of social and economic development, 3) an equitable national and international distribution of resources for health, and 4) public understanding of the political, social, economic, environmental, and biological determinants of health—understanding that would motivate people to participate in efforts to improve their health. This kind of health development contains all the ingredients necessary to act as a powerful lever for social and economic development in general.

Will these strategies make any difference, or will they have the same fate as earlier well-meant but ill-placed development efforts? It is encouraging that this report, whose authors independently pose and address this same question, points toward a positive answer. The evidence suggests that certain types of intervention to bring about health and nutrition improvements *can* make a substantial difference. The authors make a very useful contribution by bringing together—and assessing the findings of—existing social and economic analyses of ten major efforts to provide health and nutrition care in the manner supported by the Alma-Ata Declaration. The report illustrates *how* the poverty circle can be broken—how people can be helped to extricate themselves from the vicious circle of poverty, disease, malnutrition, high death rates, illiteracy, unemployment, and family growth in excess of family economic capacity.

The ten projects described—located in different national settings in several continents—make it clear, each in its own way, that hard and fast rules cannot be universally applied. The reason for the success of an intervention cannot be pinned down to any single component of a strategy. What stands out, however, is that the motivation of those involved, their understanding of the social forces at work, and their emphasis on carrying out the projects with a high degree of managerial efficiency were at least as important as the substantive content of the intervention. The authors have wisely used infant and child mortality as an indication of effectiveness. Unlike the gross national product, which can rise significantly as a result of a major improvement in the economic status of a country's elite, the infant mortality rate can only decline substantially as a result of improving the lot of the total population. Indeed, one of the striking factors in the success of these projects was that they achieved wide coverage of the populations they served.

Most significant were the annual per capita costs of the projects, which varied from about $1.50 to $7.50, including both capital and recurring expenditures. As the authors point out, these were about 0.5 per cent to 2 per cent of the annual per capita gross national product of the countries concerned, and this level of expenditure was very close to the levels of health expenditures reported for most developing countries. Such levels of expenditure on health are extremely modest by any standards, and they are much lower than the percentage of the GNP spent on health in the affluent countries. In absolute terms, these expenditures are miniscule in comparison with those in the affluent countries.

It is of particular interest to note that in these ten cases, *family* expenditures on health were substantial—often exceeding *government* expenditures. This illustrates that self-reliance is a feasible goal for developing countries. At the same time, the affluent countries have heavy obligations to transfer resources, as part of the program for the "new international economic order," to help the developing countries to "take off" along the runway that leads to self-reliance.

The types of intervention employed in these ten projects—wide population coverage, effective social as well as technical training of health personnel, and extensive employment of auxiliary and community health workers—are all components of the new approach to health development based on primary health care that was adopted in the Alma-Ata Declaration.

It is most encouraging to note in the authors' conclusions that interventions *can* make a difference. I interpret these successes to result from social interventions aiming to foster genuine human development and not merely economic growth as such, which may tend only to make the rich richer and the poor poorer. The authors have shown how a *combination* of factors—the determination to solve problems, the setting of goals, the striving to reach these goals by increasing people's social awareness, and the liberation of the physical and intellectual energy of people through improvements in their health—does make an essential difference. This suggests that health *can* be a lever for social and economic development at as low a cost as between 0.5 per cent and 2 per cent of the GNP!

In this era of cynicism and double talk about increases in official development assistance when aid in reality is decreasing, or about establishing a "new international economic order" when entrenched positions dominate rather than constructive dialogue, it is useful to show that socioeconomic development itself is the real objective—and not just a smokescreen for economic growth.

In agreeing with the conclusions of this report, I should like to stress the need for large-scale application of its findings. We are beyond the stage of timid groping for new solutions. The time has come for dynamic applications that include social and economic analyses as part of health systems research but that go far beyond this research. For sight must never be lost of the purpose of these interventions, which is to improve human life rather than to prove the superiority of any one method of intervention. This type of intervention research is in reality a constant striving for better ways of extricating the poor from their poverty and the sick from their sickness, and of leading to a progressively improved quality of life for all the people of the world.

This report, in spite of its apparent modesty, should serve to strengthen our conviction that it is possible to attain an acceptable level of health for all by the end of this century. It should highlight to the world community the urgency of adopting "health for all by the year 2000" as *the* social goal for the end of this century. It should heighten our determination to strive to reach that goal in the spirit of the Declaration of Alma-Ata. It should dispel doubts among donor agencies and inspire them to give direct support to efforts for health development as part of social and economic development—not as a charity, but in a spirit of enlightened self-interest. Finally, my personal hope is that it will also strengthen WHO's own appeal to the leaders of the world to use health as a lever for socioeconomic development and peace.

Interventions *can* make a difference—provided that they help women and men, who must be the subjects and not just the objects of development, to help themselves.

can health and nutrition interventions make a difference?

introduction

The Social and Economic Context of Intervention Efforts

Malnutrition and poor health are so clearly elements of the larger syndrome of poverty in the developing world that they are destined to remain in distressing evidence for as long as poverty itself continues to exist. Our increasing understanding of the complex interactions among the many components of this syndrome—poor nutrition, high mortality, widespread unemployment, lack of education, high birth rates, and others—has led to a growing awareness that all of these elements require attention if significant progress is to be made with respect to any one of them, or with respect to poverty as a whole.

Thus improvements in nutrition and health conditions will be strongly influenced by progress in overcoming the many other manifestations of poverty; and if little headway can be made toward improvements in such things as literacy, employment, and food availability, the prospects for the eventual achievement of adequate nutritional levels and acceptable health conditions for the world's poor will be limited. Given enough time, in fact, improvements in the economic and social environments in which the poor now live would probably by themselves suffice to overcome at least the worst aspects of malnutrition and poor health as well as the other manifestations of poverty.

But to rely on social and economic progress alone is not necessarily the best strategy. Conventional development efforts oriented toward overall economic growth have proven unusually slow in bringing about improvements in nutrition and health, as well as in fulfilling other basic needs. Recognition of this, coupled with an appreciation of the alternate approaches and technologies available, leads to a strong sense that there is no need to wait—that conventional development programs can be supplemented by many other ways of meeting the needs of the poor, such as village-based, "trickle-up" development strategies; consumer-oriented agricultural production and distribution policies; and direct intervention efforts to deal with nutrition, health, education, and other social problems.

Can Interventions Make a Difference?

Direct interventions have long been especially appealing to those concerned with nutrition and health problems. For one thing, the underlying logic seems so simple. If people are hungry, why not give them food? If they are ill, why not treat them? General development is of course important. But it takes time, and people are hungry and dying *now*. Why wait for years to increase agricultural output or to improve income distribution? Why insist on complex and indirect strategies when it is possible to meet obvious needs quickly, simply, and directly?

Also, direct help is gratifying. The poor obviously need and generally welcome subsidized food and medical care. Those providing care understandably find a great deal of satisfaction in helping fill such obvious needs, and their own psychic need to be helpful and appreciated is often best fulfilled by visible, concrete projects. In addition, the continuing need of health and nutrition program operators to mobilize political and financial support is best served by having specific discrete programs to which they can point as proof that they are doing something to help "solve" problems.

In recent years, though, the efficacy of direct intervention efforts has increasingly come into question. It has been found, for example, that when a child's diet is inadequate in calories, high-protein supplements intended to aid the child's growth are instead utilized by its body for energy—which can be equally well obtained through much less expensive foods. Also, when other members of the family are hungry too, as is almost always the case, the extra food provided is likely to be shared by all rather than allocated to the intended beneficiaries. The infections that may impair food absorption are often resistant to Western drug therapy; even when they do respond in the clinic or hospital, they are likely to recur once the children return to their unprotected home environments. In sum. the effectiveness of interventions seems limited unless everyone can get enough to eat and unless the overall environment can be improved—objectives whose achievement lies far beyond the intent or capacity of even the most ambitious direct health and nutrition intervention programs.

Of equally serious concern is the possibility that direct interventions may even be counterproductive. Significant and lasting improvements in health and nutritional conditions require social and economic changes that can be brought about only when the poorest perceive opportunities for changing their lives and have greater access to the productive resources necessary for them to do so. Intervention programs that increase the dependence of villagers on local power structures or on outside assistance—instead of increasing their potential productivity or contributing to a more equitable distribution of resources—work against the establishment of the capability and the sense of self-reliance that are vital for change.

Few would deny that there are rational grounds for many of these criticisms. But are the criticisms so convincing as to rule out any place at all for direct attacks on malnutrition and poor health? Or do some types of direct interventions still deserve a place—perhaps even an important place—in development strategies concerned with poverty, malnutrition, and poor health?

2

a focus on field experiments

The Rationale

An answer to such questions about the effectiveness of direct interventions obviously requires a look at the record—an assessment of just how effective such efforts have been in improving nutritional and health status.

Unfortunately, however, the record is often incomplete and difficult to interpret, especially with respect to the large-scale efforts that are of greatest potential interest. Overall national experiences are difficult to assess because of data limitations, and because of difficulties in sorting out the many interacting factors that influence nutrition and health trends. Assessments of other large-scale service programs are occasionally more enlightening but still have serious limitations. As one reviewer recently observed, the evaluation of such programs has been, "sadly neglected. . . . Only a minority of the 201 nutrition programs surveyed by the Harvard Institute of International Development systematically evaluated cost or nutritional-status impact data."[1] "We were amazed," reported another review team, "at how little competent work has been done in the evaluation of nutrition intervention directed towards remedying protein-energy malnutrition in preschool children."[2] A World Health Organization review has found the situation equally unsatisfactory with respect to the effective evaluation of health care programs. "Since 1934, several studies—at least 5 of them of major importance—have been carried out to evaluate the improvement of health resulting from a particular [community health center] programme. . . . With the possible exception of an investigation carried out in Ethiopia, these studies have been fairly inclusive."[3]

---

[1] James Austin et al., "Nutrition Intervention Assessment and Guidelines," report to the United Nations ACC Sub-Committee on Nutrition, June 1978, p. 15. (Mimeographed.)

[2] Jean-Pierre Habicht and William P. Butz, "Measurement of Health and Nutrition Effects of Large-Scale Intervention Projects," paper prepared for the Conference on the Measurement of the Impact of Nutrition and Related Health Programs in Latin America, Panama City, Panama, August 1-4, 1977, p. 24.

[3] Milton I. Roemer, *Evaluation of Community Health Centres,* Public Health Papers, No. 48 (Geneva: World Health Organization, 1972), p. 29. Of the studies considered major, two suggested that health center programs had not significantly affected mortality; one found that the health center had influenced mortality; two were too poorly executed to permit any conclusion to be drawn.

Not all types of interventions, it should be noted, have been as inadequately evaluated as the general primary health and nutrition care that is under consideration here, for an extensive body of literature exists with respect to the effectiveness of more specific disease-control programs. The contribution of malaria control to mortality reduction, for

This lack of adequate data about results makes it difficult to get a clear overall sense of what has been accomplished by large-scale service efforts. Few such programs have attempted to gather outcome data; even where attempts have been made, the resulting data have rarely been adequate for valid analyses. The few capable evaluations that have been carried out have concentrated primarily on specific aspects of nutritional status, particularly physical growth, without providing a broader perspective on changes in overall health conditions.

Difficulties such as these preclude the formulation of policy conclusions based on experience with national or other large-scale intervention efforts. We must look instead to the numerous relatively well organized and controlled field experiments that have provided nutrition and health services to limited populations in low-income rural areas during the past twenty-five years. Although the broader relevance of such small and careful projects may be challenged, only among them are to be found the careful records necessary for policy-relevant evaluations.

The approach adopted here, then, is to examine and summarize the experience of those field projects with the minimally adequate data needed for an assessment of their effectiveness in alleviating nutritional inadequacies and in improving health. The principal indicator examined is child health, as reflected in infant and child mortality rates, supplemented by data on physical growth when available. Mortality rates were selected primarily for practical reasons. While the use of a broader definition of health status incorporating morbidity as well as mortality considerations would be preferable, the data available from these projects are not adequate for this to be a workable approach. For all their insufficiencies, mortality data are much more frequently available, more often used, and better understood.

The focus on the health of only infants and children and not of adults was also dictated by that of the projects reviewed. It is defensible on substantive as well pragmatic grounds. Few would deny that adults are entitled to good health. But if priorities are to be established—as they must be, especially when resources are as scarce as they are in the developing world—there are several reasons for believing that infants and children merit special attention. A disproportionately large percentage of total deaths occurs at these young ages.[4] Moreover, developing-developed country inequities are much greater with re-

example, has been the topic of a great deal of sophisticated work. For an introduction to this literature, see the items cited in R. H. Gray, "The Decline of Mortality in Ceylon and the Demographic Effects of Mortality Control," *Population Studies*, Vol. 28, No. 2 (July 1974): 205-29. Another example of a subject that has received careful attention is the influence of schistosomiasis control on economic development, as discussed in Burton A. Weisbrod *et al., Disease and Economic Development* (Madison: University of Wisconsin Press, 1973). The impact of water supply on health is also well covered by the studies cited in Robert J. Saunders and Jeremy J. Warford, *Village Water Supply: Economics and Policy in the Developing World,* A World Bank Research Publication (Baltimore: Johns Hopkins University Press for World Bank, 1976).

[4] In the typical developing country, over one third of all deaths occur among children under five years of age. In the industrialized countries, the comparable figure is normally well under 5 per cent. Ansley J. Coale and Paul Demeny, *Regional Model Life Tables and Stable Populations* (Princeton, N.J.: Princeton University Press, 1966).

spect to infants and children than with respect to adults.[5] And in view of what is known about the importance of early childhood development for effective physical and intellectual performance in later life, infant and child nutrition and health efforts may well be the most effective way of improving adult well-being as well.

Given our increased understanding of and interest in the implications of the interactions between nutrition and infection, this review also provided an opportunity to examine the results of attempts to apply these theoretical concepts in field programs. The selection of projects combining "nutrition" and "health" inputs in different ways made it possible to compare the impact of different approaches to this crucial complex of factors. The fact that some of the projects provided family planning as well as nutrition and health services also permitted estimation of the utility of fertility reduction efforts undertaken in conjunction with nutrition and health interventions.

Ten Projects Selected for Review

The application of this approach led to the selection of ten projects that both tried systematically to reduce infant and child mortality in poor rural areas and kept records adequate to permit conclusions to be drawn about their accomplishments.[6] Six of the projects were also concerned with the physical growth of children, and four sought to promote family planning acceptance and fertility reduction.

It should be noted that the projects that had the best records available and that were therefore selected for review are not necessarily those that accomplished the most. The use of data adequacy as a basis for inclusion introduced a significant bias in favor of projects incorporating the concept of the scientific method—and probably other Western social and political outlooks as well. Whether this approach involved a bias toward projects that performed more effectively than others is unclear. The possibility certainly exists that the bias lies in the other direction, for many impressive projects have been executed without much heed to data collection. For example, the data-adequacy criterion eliminates from consideration all but one (Jamkhed) of the several interesting community-based efforts described in the World Health Organization's volume *Health by the People;*[7] it precludes coverage of the Palghar and Miraj projects in India, the Huehuetenango and La Pasion projects in Guatemala; the Savar

---

[5] Infant mortality rates are 8-10 times higher, and child mortality rates 30-50 times higher, in the typical developing country (where life expectancy is 55 years) than in the typical economically advanced nation (life expectancy of 75 years). The differential declines steadily with increasing age—developing-country mortality rates being "only" two or three times as high as those of the developed world for people 50-55 years of age. Ibid.

[6] Appendix A contains the list of project features considered relevant for evaluation purposes which guided this review. The available information on which the review is based—published and unpublished project reports, and correspondence and conversations with project directors supplemented by information from others familiar with the projects reviewed and from the authors' personal experience—was not adequate to permit full coverage of all items on the list.

[7] Kenneth W. Newell, ed., *Health by the People* (Geneva: World Health Organization, 1975).

and Brac projects in Bangladesh; Project Piaxtla in Mexico;[8] and it prevents discussion of India's long experience with village-based approaches to improved health inspired by the work of Mahatma Gandhi. Thus while the projects surveyed were doubtless much more effective than the average developing-country health program, there is no basis for asserting that they were the most successful to have been undertaken.

Several other well-known projects in the Western scientific tradition were omitted from this review because their final results were not yet available. Among them were projects undertaken in Lampang, Thailand; Deschapelles, Haiti; and Bohol, Philippines.[9] The otherwise well-documented Candelaria, Colombia, and Danfa, Ghana, projects were excluded for lack of adequate mortality data.

In chronological order, the ten projects covered are:

Many Farms, U.S.A.: an Arizona Navajo reservation project begun in 1956 by the Cornell University Medical School. It was one of the first attempts to apply the technologically advanced, physician-based, curative medical orientation of "modern scientific" medicine to a traditional, low-income population in an environment startlingly similar to that of many areas of the developing world today.

Rural Guatemala I: the first of two major village-level intervention studies undertaken by the Nutrition Institute of Central America and Panama (INCAP). Launched in 1959, it was the first effort to explore systematically the interaction between nutrition and infection, providing nutrition supplements in one village, health care in another, and using a third village as a control.

Imesi, Nigeria: an outreach service effort of the prominent Wesley Guild Mission Hospital, initiated around 1960. It was this project that originated the "under-fives" clinic concept, featuring frequent comprehensive care for infants and young children and the regular weighing of infants as a means of monitoring their nutritional status and identifying those in need of special attention.

---

[8] In addition to the chapters in Newell's *Health by the People*, the descriptions of these and other projects can be found in Mary V. Ammel, "Rural Health Promoters' Program: Fifteen Years' Experience in Community Health, Huehuetenango, Guatemala," paper presented at the Second Annual Conference of the International Federation of Public Health Associations, Halifax, Nova Scotia, May 23, 1978, mimeographed; Zafarulla Chowdhury, "The Mother and Child in Bangladesh: A View from the People's Health Centre," *Les Carnets d'Enfance/Assignment Children*, Vol. 33 (January-March 1976); Eric R. Ram, "Integrated Health Services: The Miraj Project in India," *Les Carnets d'Enfance/Assignment Children*, Vol. 39 (July-September 1977); P.M. Shah *et al.*, "Communitywide Surveillance of 'At Risk' Under-Fives in Need of Special Care," *Environmental Child Health* (June 1976): 103-7; David Bradford Werner, "Health Care and Human Dignity: A Subjective Look at Community-Based Rural Health Programs in Latin America," Hesperian Foundation, Palo Alto, California, 1976, mimeographed; Working Group on Rural Medical Care, "Delivery of Primary Care by Medical Auxiliaries: Techniques of Use and Analysis of Benefits Achieved in Some Rural Villages in Guatemala, " in Pan American Health Organization, *Medical Auxiliaries: Proceedings of A Symposium Held During the Twelfth Meeting of the PAHO Advisory Committee on Medical Research June 25, 1973*, PAHO Scientific Publication No. 278, pp. 24-37.

[9] The initial findings of the Bohol project have since been published in Beth S. Atkins, consulting ed., "The MCH/FP Approach: Report from Bohol, the Philippines," *Studies in Family Planning*, Vol. 10, No. 6/7 (June/July 1979), pp. 187-216. These findings are briefly summarized, and their implications for the conclusions of this review noted, in footnote 21 below.

Northern Peru: a five-year experiment that sought to determine the nutrition and health effects of high-protein food supplements distributed to entire families living in villages on a sugar plantation. It was conducted by the research department of Lima's British-American Hospital.

Etimesgut, Turkey: a pilot project to test the effectiveness of a set of medical and family planning services that could be offered by a national health program for rural regions. The project was implemented, beginning in 1965, by the Hacettepe University Institute of Community Medicine in an agricultural area near Ankara.

Narangwal, India: a further field exploration of the interaction between nutrition and infection. Conducted in the state of Punjab from 1968 to 1973 by the Johns Hopkins School of Hygiene and Public Health in collaboration with the Indian Council of Medical Research, the project provided nutrition supplements and education in one area, health care in another, and both nutrition and health services in a third. A fourth group of villages, with no services, was a control area. A parallel project tested different approaches to family planning service delivery.

Rural Guatemala II: the second of INCAP's village intervention projects, carried out between 1969 and 1977 in four Guatemalan communities different from those included in Rural Guatemala I. The project's objective was to study the influence of nutrition supplements on child development, and the impact of medical services provided by health auxiliaries on health conditions.

Jamkhed, India: a village-level service project established in 1971 by two Indian physicians in a small town 400 kilometers southeast of Bombay in the state of Maharashtra. The project, which features efforts to involve local community leaders in its design and implementation, provides a wide range of nutrition, health, and family planning services.

Hanover, Jamaica: a pilot service project initiated in 1973 by the Cornell University Medical College, the University of the West Indies, and the Jamaican government. The approach has featured regular nutrition monitoring and nutrition education by community health aides.

Kavar, Iran: a pilot health service and nutrition education project of the Pahlavi University Department of Community Medicine, begun in 1973 in a rural area near Shiraz. The objective of the project, is to test the applicability of a paramedical "barefoot doctor" approach to rural Iran. Maternal health and family planning services have been among those offered.

These projects covered populations ranging from 2,000 (Many Farms) to 65,000 (Hanover), with the number of people served by most of them lying toward the lower end of the range. The majority of the projects included both nutrition and health components, but some did not: the Northern Peru project provided only fortified food supplements; Many Farms and Etimesgut offered only medical care. Those projects that did incorporate both nutrition and health services displayed a considerable variety of approaches.

This heterogeneity resulted in part from wide differences in the economic, social, and cultural settings, in part from differences in program objectives. Projects such as Rural Guatemala I and II and Northern Peru were primarily research efforts designed to produce data for scientific study. Etimesgut, Hanover, and Kavar were pilot projects, undertaken to test health care approaches with potential for large-scale application. Imesi and Jamkhed, on the other hand, were health care programs primarily concerned with providing the best possible services in the project area and only secondarily interested in the wider implications of their approaches for nationwide health efforts or academic thinking. All of the programs included elements of more than one of these orientations. Some, such as Many Farms and Narangwal, incorporated so many that they refuse to fit neatly into any single category.

The state of the art prevailing at the time when the various intervention efforts began was another source of variation. The Many Farms project was started in the mid-1950s, before the role of nutrition was widely appreciated; the project reports hardly mention the term. The project's emphasis was instead on high-technology medicine, supplemented by the input of academically qualified anthropologists, who were considered the best source of advice on how to adapt the technological approach to a traditional culture. The Northern Peru project of the early 1960s featured the use of fish protein concentrate, then of particular interest in nutrition circles, to enrich the dietary staple. The Narangwal project, developed in the late 1960s, was a field test of the operational implications of the synergistic relationship between infection and nutrition—a relationship that had been explored for the first time under field conditions only a few years before in the Rural Guatemala I project. The Jamkhed and Kavar projects reflected the interest in greater community involvement that arose in the early 1970s in response to the accomplishments apparently achieved in a number of socialist states, notably China and Cuba, through emphasis on rural development. Kavar was a conscious effort to adapt the Chinese "barefoot doctor" approach to Iranian conditions.

In brief, each project had its own distinctive characteristics, reflecting local conditions and needs, the predilections and orientation of its leaders, and the temper of the time at which it was undertaken. Yet the projects shared two important characteristics that justify grouping them together for a common review: all sought in one way or another to move out of the hospital toward the village in an effort to deal more effectively with problems of infant and child health and nutrition, and all tried to measure the success of their efforts.

8

the impact of the interventions on infant and child mortality, physical growth, and fertility

The Individual Project Findings

What did these projects accomplish? From the available reports, supplemented by conversations and correspondence with the project leaders, it is possible to prepare a brief summary of each project's results.[10] The findings presented below and in Tables 1 and 2 (pp. 14-17) are principally those directly relevant to infant and child mortality and, to a lesser extent, to physical growth and fertility. Many of the projects contained other components, such as studies of mental development, whose outcomes are not reported. Also, as will be discussed in greater detail later, the focus on mortality reduction omits possible unanticipated, and thus unmeasured, effects of the projects on other aspects of village life—on social and economic structures, for example, and on the villagers' relations with authorities from outside the village.

Many Farms, U.S.A. During the five years of the project, infant mortality declined from 116 to 76 (per 1,000 live births). For a variety of reasons, however, such as small sample size, lack of controls, and erratic year-to-year changes, the significance of the decline is unclear. The investigators concluded that the project had not had a significant impact on overall mortality levels—a conclusion that gave rise to the idea of a "technologic misfit" between the modern medical approach used in the project and the diarrhea-pneumonia complex of diseases found to be dominant among the infants and children of Many Farms.[11] Data on child mortality, physical growth, and fertility were not available; nor was there information on project costs.

Rural Guatemala I. Infant mortality declined by about one third in one intervention village and by one fifth in the other, while rising slightly in the control village. The number of deaths reported in each case was small, however, and differences in earlier mortality trends raised questions about the comparability of the three villages. Child mortality rates, calculated in most cases on the basis of even fewer deaths, declined substantially in all three villages—about 30 and 50 per cent in the two intervention villages and about 40 per cent in the control village. The numerous complications encountered prevented the investigators from reaching what they considered to be unambiguous conclusions about the project's impact on mortality trends. Physical growth

---

[10] For a list of the reports on which the summaries are based, see the bibliography. The profiles in Appendix B report provide further detail with respect to each project.

[11] Walsh McDermott, "Modern Medicine and the Demographic-Disease Pattern of Overly Traditional Societies; A Technologic Misfit," *Journal of Medical Education*, Vol. 41 (Supplement, 1966): 137-62.

was moderately more rapid in the area served with nutrition supplements than in the other areas. Fertility and cost data were not available.

Imesi, Nigeria. Approximately five years after the project's initiation, infant mortality was 57 in Imesi, 91 in a nearby control village; the child mortality rate was 18 (per 1,000 children 1-5 years of age) in Imesi, 51 in the control village. Children in Imesi were 4-6 per cent heavier and 2-3 per cent taller than in the control village. The crude birth rate was 45 in Imesi, 43 in the control village; the general fertility rate was one third higher in Imesi than in the control village (228 compared to 171). The per capita cost was $1.50 annually, or about 2 per cent of Nigeria's yearly per capita income at the time.

Northern Peru. During the five-year study period, there was no significant difference in physical growth between the treatment and control areas. However, infant mortality averaged 48 in the treatment areas, compared to 134 in the control areas; child mortality averaged 22 in the treatment areas, 40 in the control areas. Fertility and cost data were not available.

Etimesgut, Turkey. The Etimesgut infant mortality rate fell from 142 to 72 between 1967 and 1977. The decline between 1967 and 1973 was 34 per cent (from 142 to 93), compared with a decline of 28 per cent (from 153 to 110) for Turkey as a whole. The child mortality rate fell from 59 (per 1,000 children aged 0-5) in 1967 to 37 in 1977. Information about physical growth was not available. The crude birth rate, stable at around 35 before 1969, fell steadily to 27 in 1974 and has remained at around 27-28 thereafter. The annual per capita cost was $6.50 to $7.50, or 2 per cent of the yearly per capita income in Turkey.

Narangwal, India. Infant mortality was 25 to 40 per cent lower in the three treatment areas than in the control areas; child mortality (one to three years of age) was 30 to 40 per cent lower. At 36 months of age, children in the treatment areas were 6 to 7 per cent (0.5 to 0.6 kg.) heavier and 1 to 2 per cent (0.2 to 1.3 cm.) taller than children in the control areas, with children in the nutrition care villages in general showing the most rapid growth. The annual cost of services ranged from around $0.80 per person for medical care alone to $2.00 per person for nutrition services, equal to roughly 1 to 2 per cent of India's per capita annual income at the time. In the companion family planning project, the general fertility rate fell 4 to 21 per cent in the areas that offered various combinations of family planning, health, and welfare services, compared with a 3 per cent decline in the control area.

Rural Guatemala II. Infant mortality fell by about two thirds (from around 150 to 55) and child mortality by around three fourths (from 28 to 6) within two to three years after the project's initiation—declines notably more rapid than the 5 per cent reduction in infant mortality (from 89 to 85) and the 15 per cent fall in child mortality (from 26 to 22) reported for Guatemala as a whole during approximately the same period. Children who regularly received high-protein food supplements grew 10 to 15 per cent more rapidly than children who did not. Neither fertility data nor cost figures for the nutrition component were available. The program's health component, believed by the project investigators to be responsible for most of the mortality decline, cost about $3.50 per capita annually. This figure was somewhat under 1 per cent of the Guatemalan average per capita income in 1971.

Jamkhed, India. In the relatively small sample population surveyed, infant mortality declined from 97 in 1971 to 39 in 1976, compared to 90 in the (also small) sample of the control area population covered in the 1976 survey. The crude birth rates in the same population samples were 40 in 1971 and 23 in 1976 for the experimental area, compared to 37 in 1976 for the control area. The cost was roughly estimated at $1.25 to $1.50 per person annually, or just over 1 per cent of the Indian per capita GNP in the mid-1970s. Child mortality and physical growth data were not available.

Hanover, Jamaica. In Hanover Parish, infant mortality fell from an annual average of 36 between 1970 and 1973 to 11 in 1975, compared with a decline from 26 in 1973 to 23 in 1975 in Jamaica as a whole. The child mortality rate (1-48 months of age) fell by more than one half (from 13-15 to 5-6) within a year of the program's initiation. The proportion of children who weighed less than 75 per cent of the weight expected for their age fell from 11-13 per cent to 6-7 per cent within a year of the start of the program. The investigators have tentatively established the pilot project's cost at $2.50 per child, or around $0.40 per person—about one twentieth of 1 per cent of Jamaica's annual average per capita income. Fertility data were not available.

Kavar, Iran. Two surveys taken after the project's initiation yielded estimated infant mortality rates in the treatment area 50 to 60 per cent below those found in the control area. The first, fifteen months after the project had begun, found an infant mortality rate of 65 in the treatment area, 128 in the control area. Three years later the rates recorded were 84 and 138. The crude birth rate was 40 in the treatment area and 45 in the control area according to the first survey, 37 in each area according to the second. The per person cost was estimated at $3.50 to $5.25 annually in 1975, depending upon the method of calculation used—a sum equal to roughly one half of 1 per cent of Iran's national per capita income. Data on physical growth and child mortality were not available.

General Findings

What generalizations can be drawn from the results of these individual projects?

Effectiveness. To begin with, the available data suggest strongly that declines in infant and child mortality occurred in all of the areas served by these ten projects. Most of the declines were large: on the order of one third to one half, sometimes more. And they were rapid, appearing within one to five years of the projects' initiation.

In themselves, though, such mortality declines are not necessarily significant. Infant and child mortality has been declining throughout the developing world over most of the past quarter-century—often rapidly, and without the benefit of efforts nearly as intense as those provided by the projects. The important question to be answered in assessing program effectiveness is thus not simply whether mortality declines occurred in the project areas, but whether the declines occurring there were larger than those recorded elsewhere, and whether the services offered by the projects were responsible for the difference.

For methodological reasons to be discussed later, this turns out to be extremely difficult to demonstrate conclusively. Yet there is still a very persuasive, even if not totally decisive, case to be made that mortality declines were notably more rapid in a clear majority of the ten project sites than they would have been in the projects' absence.

Some relevant information about mortality levels or trends outside the experimental areas is available for nine of the ten projects.[12] In five cases (Imesi, Rural Guatemala I, Northern Peru, Narangwal, and Kavar), the project assessments provide information about relatively comparable control areas; in one case (Jamkhed), control-area data are also available from the project reports, although the comparability of the control and experimental areas is more difficult to assess; in three (Etimesgut, Hanover, and Rural Guatemala II), the comparison is principally with national-level figures.

In seven of the nine cases for which some comparison is possible, the data suggest that infant and child mortality fell more rapidly in the project areas than in the control areas or in the nation as a whole. The two exceptions were Rural Guatemala I, where the results were ambiguous; and Etimesgut, where the declines in infant and child mortality were not sufficiently different from national trends to be clearly attributable to the services provided by the project, especially in light of Etimesgut's proximity to the urban, modernizing influences of Ankara, Turkey's capital city.

With respect to fertility, five of the ten projects provided data adequate to permit trend estimates. Four had sought consciously to lower birth rates and had provided family planning services in conjunction with nutrition and health efforts. In three of these four cases (Etimesgut, Narangwal, Jamkhed), the decline reported was substantial; in the fourth (Kavar), it was not clear whether fertility had fallen more rapidly in the treatment than in the control area. Of the six projects not providing family planning services, only one (Imesi) reported fertility data. There, a survey taken five years after the project's initiation found fertility to be higher in the treatment than in the control area.

Five of the six projects that sought to stimulate physical growth also appear to have achieved at least some results. The exception was the Northern Peru project, where no significant difference between the treatment and control populations was reported.

Costs. Seven of the ten projects provide information about the cost of their operations and accomplishments. Although estimates are often impressionistic, they were adequate to indicate that expenditures were generally modest. The annual per capita cost varied from about $0.30 to $7.50, including both capital and recurring expenditures.[13] This amounted to about 0.5-2.0 per cent of the annual per capita gross national products of the countries concerned for the years to which the cost figures refer.[14] These expenditures were very close to

---

[12] Many Farms, where extreme differences between the project area and the rest of U.S. society rendered even national-level statistics inapplicable, was the one area for which no minimally acceptable control data were available.

[13] Capital costs and recurring costs are given separately in most project reports. An annual capital cost estimation has been made by assuming a 10-20 year life for capital items, which means adding 5-10 per cent of total capital costs to the annual recurring cost to arrive at total costs. The procedure used makes little difference in the outcome, since the great majority of costs (usually 90 per cent or more) is recurring.

[14] The ranges of $0.80-$7.50 per capita annual costs and 0.5-2.0 per cent of GNP both exclude the particularly sketchy cost data available for the Hanover, Jamaica project, which suggest an annual per capita cost of $0.40, or 0.05 per cent of annual GNP.

the 0.5-3.0 per cent of GNP health expenditure levels reported by the World Bank for most developing countries. Because of the concentration of facilities in urban, relatively affluent areas, the proportion of the total population served by the more conventional systems to which the World Bank figures refer is thought to be quite small.[15] Thus, the cost per person actually served by conventional national health care systems is probably many times higher than suggested by 0.5-3.0 per cent of GNP, and consequently also much higher than the widely accessible services provided by the projects reviewed.

This is even more likely to be true when the potential role of patient fees and other local contributions to primary nutrition and health care programs is taken into account. Family health care expenditures in the developing world are substantial, often exceeding those of governments. This raises the possibility that some of the costs of expanded official primary care systems might be shifted onto families. Both of the two projects reviewed that developed primarily as service-delivery rather than as pilot-research efforts included patient fee payments as central elements in their approaches: patient fees covered about 40 per cent of Imesi's operating costs, around 75 per cent of Jamkhed's. The Jamkhed project investigators felt that, in addition to making the programs less expensive for the outside supporters, such cost-sharing would serve effectively to enhance consumer participation and responsibility.

The general comparability of the cost figures cited suggests that the conventional health and nutrition service pattern, with its inevitably limited coverage, could be replaced by the wide-coverage approaches of the projects reviewed here at little increase in overall governmental health expenditures. If it were possible to achieve on a larger scale a level of primary-care effectiveness comparable to that of these projects, such a reallocation of funds would seem likely to lead to considerable gains in both equity of coverage and overall infant and child mortality conditions. Although so drastic a reorientation is rarely likely to be feasible politically, such rough calculations suggest that placing greater reliance on the kinds of nutrition and health approaches reviewed here can be attractive from an economic as well as from a health-policy point of view.

---

[15] World Bank, *Health,* Sector Policy Paper (Washington, D.C.: World Bank, March 1975), pp. 74-75. Forty-two of the 50 developing countries listed are in this 0.5-3.0 per cent range. Five are under, three are over.

Table 1. General Characteristics and Reported Results for the Ten Projects

Location	Dates	Type of Project	Principal Services	Approximate Size of Treatment Population[a]	Reported Results: Physical Growth[b]
1. Many Farms, U.S.A.	1956-62	Research/ Pilot	Medical Services	2.000	—
2. Rural Guatemala I	1959-64	Research	Food Supplements/Medical Services	1.700	Nutrition care children 1 kg. (6%-7%) heavier, 3 cm. (2%-3%) taller than health care or control children at five years of age.
3. Imesi, Nigeria	c. 1960-	Service	Nutrition Surveillance/Medical Services	6.000	Treatment children 0.3-0.4 kg. (4%-6%) heavier, 1.5-3.0 cm. (2%-3%) taller than control children after 6-12 mos. of age.
4. Northern Peru	1962-67	Research	Food Supplements	1.800	No significant differences between treatment and control areas.
5. Etimesgut, Turkey	1965-	Pilot	Medical Services	55.000	—
6. Narangwal, India	1968-73	Research/ Pilot	Medical Services/Nutrition Supplements and Education	10.500	Treatment children 0.5-0.6 kg. (6%-7%) heavier and 0.2-1.3 cm. (0%-2%) taller than others at 36 mos. of age.
7. Rural Guatemala II	1972-77	Research	Nutrition Supplements/Medical Services	3.000	Children receiving high-protein supplements grew 10%-15% more rapidly than other children.
8. Jamkhed, India	1971-	Service	Nutrition Supplements and Education/Medical Services	40.000	—
9. Hanover, Jamaica	1973-	Pilot	Nutrition Surveillance/Medical Services	65.000	Proportion of children below 75% of expected weight for age fell from 11%-13% to 6%-7% within one year of program initiation.
10. Kavar, Iran	1973-	Pilot	Medical Services/Health and Nutrition Education	8.200	

[a]Total project population (infants, children, and adults) excluding control population, if any.

[b]Reported results, with respect both to physical growth and to mortality, are subject to the several methodological considerations discussed on pp. 25-29, in the individual project profiles in Appendix B, and in the project investigators' reports of their work.

[c]Deaths 0-12 months per 1,000 live births.

[d]Deaths per 1,000 population aged 12-60 months, except for: 1) Etimesgut, where figures are deaths 0-60 months per 1,000 population 0-60 months; 2) Narangwal, where data refer to deaths 12-36 months per 1,000 population 12-36 months; 3) Hanover, with figures covering deaths 1-48 months per 1,000 population 1-48 months.

14

	Reported Results: Infant Mortality[c]				Reported Results: Child Mortality[d]				Annual Per Capita Cost (% of per capita annual income)[e]
Before (1957)	116				—				—
After (1961)	76								
	1950-59	*1959-64*	*Change*		*1950-59*	*1959-64*	*Change*		
Health Care Area	136	88	−35%		50	34	−31%		—
Nutrition Care Area	182	146	−21%		56	24	−56%		
Control Area	186	191	+3%		81	50	−38%		
	1966/67				*1966/67*				
Treatment Area	48				18				$1.50 (2%)
Control Area	91				51				
	1962-67				*1962-67*				
Treatment Area	48				22				—
Control Area	134				40				
	1967	*1973*	*1977*	*Change 1967-73*	*1967*	*1977*			
Treatment Area	142	93	73	−34%	59	37			$6.50-$7.50 (1.5%-2.0%)
Turkey	153	110		−28%					
	1970-73 (Average)				*1970-73 (Average)*				
Nutrition Care Area	97				11				$.080-$2.00 (1.5%-2.0%)
Medical Care Area	70				11				
Nutrition/Medical Care Area	81				13				
Control Area	128				19				
	1969	*1970*	*1970/72*	*Change*	*1969*	*1970*	*1970/72*	*Change*	
Treatment Area	@150		@55	−63	28		6	−79%	$3.50 (0.75%-1.0%)
Guatemala	89	85		−4%	26	22		−15%	
	1971	*1976*			*1971*	*1976*			
Treatment Area	97	39			97	39			$1.25-$1.50 (1.00%-1.25%)
Control Area		90				90			
	1970-73	*1973*	*1975*	*Change*	*1972-74*	*1973-75*			
Treatment Area	36		11	−77%	13-15	5-6			$0.40 (.05%)
Jamaica		26	23	−12%					
	1975	*1977/78*			$3.50-$5.35 (0.4%-0.5%)				
Treatment Area	65	84							—
Control Area	128	138							

[e]Recurring plus capital costs (with annual capital cost estimated at 5-10 per cent of total stated total capital expenditure). Data for Hanover refer to predecessor Elderslie pilot project; cost figures for the Hanover project itself are not available. The Elderslie cost figures are currently under review, with a significant upward revision likely. The GNP calculations are based on figures from the appropriate volume of the World Bank's *World Tables* for that year or those years to which the cost figures refer. Guatemala II villages costs refer to medical component only. Figures for nutrition costs are not available.

Table 2. Family Planning/Fertility Reduction Interests of the Ten Projects

Location	Emphasis on Family Planning Fertility Reduction
1. Many Farms, U.S.A.	None reported.
2. Rural Guatemala I	None reported.
3. Imesi, Nigeria	None reported.
4. Northern Peru	None reported.
5. Etimesgut, Turkey	The effective provision of family planning services in the context of a maternal and child health program constituted a leading project objective.
6. Narangwal, India	A separate population project, offering several integrated packages combining different health and nutrition service components with family planning, was operated in parallel with the nutrition and health intervention project. The population project served a total of approximately 21,800 people residing in villages near those covered by the nutrition and health study.
7. Rural Guatemala II	None reported.
8. Jamkhed, India	The provision of contraceptive services was an integral part of the project's maternal and child health program.
9. Hanover, Jamaica	None reported.
10. Kavar, Iran	The provision of contraceptive services was an integral part of the project's maternal and child health program.

[a]Figures for family planning service and education area and control area are as adjusted downward by the investigators (from −27.4% and −12.4%, respectively) to account for the absence of one vital statistics data source in each area. The investigators suggest a

Reported Results: Contraceptive Acceptance	Reported Results: Fertility
	Crude Birth Rate 1966-67: *General Fertility Rate 1966-67:* Treatment Area 45 Treatment Area 228 Control Area 43 Control Area 171

Reported Results: Contraceptive Acceptance	Reported Results: Fertility
Currently Using or Have Ever Used IUD: 1967 14% 1973 41% *Currently Using or Have Ever Used Pill:* 1967 7% 1973 23% *Currently Using or Ever Using Any Method:* 1967 57% 1973 74%	*Crude Birth Rate:* 1967 35.1 1969 35.4 1972 29.5 1974 26.9 1977 28.4 *Total Fertility Rate:* 1967 4.95 1969 4.94 1972 3.97 1974 3.68 1977 —

Current Users of Contraception After 1¾ and 4½ Years of Service:
Family Planning Service/Women's
  Service/Child Care Area   22% 34%
Family Planning Service/Women's
  Service Area   25% 41%
Family Planning Service/Child Care
  Area   27% —
Family Planning Service and Education
  Area   30% —
Control Area   — —
	Percentage Decline in General Fertility Rate between 1969-70 and 1973:
	Family Planning Service/Women's
	  Service/Child Care Area −16.2
	Family Planning Service/Women's
	  Service Area −18.4
	Family Planning Service/Child Care
	  Area −4.1
	Family Planning Service and Education
	  Area[a] −20.9
	Control Area[a] −2.7

Percentage of Eligible Couples Practicing Contraception: Treatment Area, 1971 2.5% Treatment Area, 1976 50.5% Control Area, 1976 10.0%	*Crude Birth Rate:* Treatment Area, 1971 40 Treatment Area, 1976 23 Control Area, 1976 37
	Crude Birth Rate: Treatment Area 40.2 Control Area 44.9

further downward revision in the family planning service and education area (to −12.9% for 1971/72—1973) to reflect data reliability problems for 1969/70 and 1971.

factors contributing to program effectiveness

Specific Components

Identifying the most effective components of the intervention programs is no easy task. Although all the projects reviewed were based on nutrition and/or health services of some kind, those that appear to have been effective seem at first glance to have little else in common beyond their apparent effectiveness. The Northern Peru project, for example, had a significant impact on mortality through take-home food supplements alone, while the equally effective Kavar project paid only limited attention to nutrition and concentrated instead on basic medical services. As will be discussed in greater detail below, the evidence is not clear enough to support an assertion that any one of the varied programmatic approaches employed showed itself to be inherently superior to the others.

Amid the diversity, though, several specific innovative measures or features of the different projects seemed to stand out as particularly effective whenever they were employed—and thus to be worthy of further attention. In addition, the project findings permit an exploration of the effectiveness of some of the more traditional components of nutrition and health intervention programs.

Maternal Nutrition Supplements. The value of nutrition programs for expectant mothers was explored most extensively in the Rural Guatemala II project, where the impact of maternal food supplements on birth weights and death rates was impressively documented. Heavier birth weights were strongly associated with lower death rates. The findings at Narangwal were similar: iron, folic acid, and food supplements for expectant mothers seem to have been associated with a significant decline in mortality at very young ages. Indeed, although efforts to improve maternal nutrition through services providing iron, folic acid, food, and nutrition education were a relatively small part of the Narangwal project, this component seems to have been a particularly effective means of averting early infant deaths. Increased maternal food intake, with its possible influence on both birth weight and maternal lactation capacity, has also been suggested as an explanation for the Northern Peru project's otherwise puzzling findings that food given to entire families helped to reduce infant mortality without contributing to more rapid physical growth among children.

The fact that maternal nutrition was given explicit attention in only a few of the projects is a reflection of the relatively recent appreciation of its importance. In fact, much of our understanding of the importance of maternal nutrition is derived from the findings of the Rural Guatemala II project, which became available only after even the most recent of the projects reviewed already had been initiated. Similarly, in the projects covered, few attempts were made to alter breastfeeding practices through either maternal nutrition supplements or maternal nutrition education.

Maternal Immunization against Tetanus. Concerted efforts to immunize pregnant women against tetanus were part of the Narangwal and Rural Guatemala II projects because of the effective protection of the newborn through placentally transmitted immunity. In Narangwal, an early survey showed that tetanus was responsible for almost 20 per cent of neonatal deaths. Project personnel were able to immunize 87 per cent of the mothers and estimated that at least 80 per cent of the potential deaths from neonatal tetanus were thereby averted. Tetanus immunization for prospective mothers also appears to have made a significant contribution to infant and child mortality declines in the Rural Guatemala II project.[16] Such experiences commend the immunization of mothers as a particularly promising component of health and nutrition programs in other communities where neonatal tetanus remains a problem.

Nutrition Monitoring. Nutrition monitoring was pioneered with considerable success at Imesi and later refined with equally encouraging results in the Narangwal and Hanover projects. In all three, growth monitoring based on regular anthropometric measurements of children in the project area facilitated the early identification of infants and young children who failed to gain weight or actually lost weight and, as a consequence, were subject to increased mortality risk. Nutrition supplementation, medical treatment, and nutrition education efforts could then be focused on these children and their families.

Regular anthropometric measurements also served in these programs as an important tool in alerting mothers to the retarded growth of their children, thereby encouraging improved feeding practices. In some situations, as in the Hanover project, the demonstration effect of these measurements was felt to be even more important than the nutrition supplements or nutrition education provided in reducing young child mortality and malnutrition. Thus, in communities where social or cultural factors play a greater role than absolute resource inadequacy in the etiology of malnutrition, nutrition monitoring appears to have the potential for a significant impact on mortality even in the absence of more expensive and more difficult to implement components such as nutrition supplementation or education.

Widespread Coverage. In contrast to the achievement of conventional official health services in most developing countries which reach only 15-20 per cent of the population in need,[17] the coverage of the projects reviewed was

---

[16] Other field experimentation also illustrates the potentially important role of tetanus immunization. In a well-known Haiti study, for example, the previously high incidence of tetanus declined by nearly 90 per cent after an immunization program. Warren L. Berggren, "Administration and Evaluation of Rural Health Services: I. A Tetanus Control Program in Haiti," *The American Journal of Tropical Medicine and Hygiene,* Vol. 23, No. 5 (September 1974): 936-49.

[17] Among the several WHO publications suggesting that no more than 20 per cent or so of developing-country populations have access to modern health services is Newell, *Health by the People,* p. ix. The World Bank *Health,* Sector Policy Paper, pp. 35-38, contains a further discussion of the limitations in the coverage of traditional developing-country health services.

remarkably complete. In many cases, almost all of the target population was surveyed at the project's outset and received services regularly thereafter.

At Imesi, for example, over 95 per cent of the village children were enrolled in the project, and they were seen once every two weeks on the average. In Northern Peru, more than 95 per cent of the families consumed the full food ration provided during the life of the project. The Hanover project screened over 90 per cent of children in the project area. Those projects offering immunizations reported reaching 80 per cent or more of the eligible children.

The vigorous outreach efforts responsible for such widespread coverage in many of the projects also appear to have reduced the social disparities in access to services that often typify more passive nutrition and health activities. The Jamkhed project, for example, sent its health teams to the villages in the early mornings so that they might be more easily available to serve poor families before they had to leave for the fields.

Unless services reach those in need, even the best-conceived primary health and nutrition care programs can obviously have little impact on mortality. Thus, as the experience of these projects demonstrates, the development of plans for getting services to the people is as important as are decisions concerning which services should be offered.

Greater Reliance on Paramedical Personnel. Several of the projects experimented with ways of giving more responsibility to paramedical personnel for the provision of simple curative services in order to facilitate broader population coverage. The Narangwal project attributed the considerable reduction achieved in deaths from diarrheal and respiratory diseases to reliance on family health workers to diagnose these problems, to administer penicillin as necessary, and to show mothers how to administer oral rehydration procedures. The Kavar, Jamkhed, Hanover, and Rural Guatemala II projects also relied heavily on paramedical personnel to deliver services—all with considerable apparent impact on infant and child mortality.

Effective Training Programs. Several project reports emphasized the importance of effective training. Although important differences existed and full details were not always available, the most successful training programs (such as those of the Kavar, Narangwal, and Rural Guatemala II projects) shared several common features. They were developed by health professionals thoroughly familiar with local problems, having themselves dealt with such problems under field conditions. Formal training was usually brief and carried out close to the homes of the trainees. Greater emphasis was placed on active, on-the-job training guided by experienced workers who were themselves capable of performing the required tasks within the constraints imposed by local conditions. And the initial training was reinforced with intensive continuing education based on frequent and regular meetings of field workers and supervisors.

When field-oriented training of this sort was not provided, difficulties often developed. At Kavar, for example, the project investigators found that an initial overemphasis on formal training led village health workers to become interested primarily in providing curative medical services, to the detriment of preventive and public health activities. Their finding—which illustrates the kind of important information that can be provided by a careful monitoring of program activities—resulted in changes in the village health worker training program that were of great value to the project.

The most effective training programs were usually closely linked to personnel systems that facilitated effective utilization of the training received. Among other things, such systems featured the careful development and application of workable job descriptions, the provision of continuing and supportive supervision, and the delegation of an adequate degree of responsibility.

Other Nutrition and Health Measures. Not surprisingly, the ten projects effectively confirmed the importance of improved nutrition for reductions in infant and child mortality. Data from the Narangwal project, for example, showed that each 10 per cent decrease in weight for age brought an exponential increase in the probability of death. A child under three years of age weighing between 60 per cent and 70 per cent of the Harvard weight-for-age standard was ten times more likely to die than a child weighing over 80 per cent of the standard. All but one of the seven more successful projects contained nutrition components of some kind, compared with only one of the three earlier, less obviously successful ones.

Several specific nutrition program components also appear to have made notable contributions. A pair of particularly promising nutrition approaches—nutrition supplements for expectant and nursing mothers and nutrition monitoring—have already been identified. In addition, nutrition supplements for infants and children seem to have been effective in reducing mortality in the Northern Peru project, and to have had an important impact in the Narangwal and Rural Guatemala I and II projects.

To state that nutrition interventions as a class are inherently superior to health interventions as a class would, however, require much more solid evidence than these studies provide. As noted, a number of health measures—maternal immunization against tetanus, increased reliance on paramedical personnel—were also very effective in helping reduce mortality. Child immunization programs were widely used, with apparent impact. All but one of the seven more obviously successful projects included some kind of a health component in addition to a nutrition element. And under some circumstances. the health interventions employed appear to have been more effective than the particular nutrition components used. At Narangwal, for example, the cost of preventing an infant or child death was lower in the medical care area than in the nutrition care area for all but the very youngest age groups. And the leaders of the Rural Guatemala II project attributed 70 per cent of the observed mortality decline to their health interventions, only 30 per cent to their nutrition efforts. Such experiences illustrate the difficulty, even in carefully managed programs, of reaching enough needy children with enough additional food at the right time to realize fully the inherent potential of a nutrition supplement program.

All this argues for pragmatism and flexibility. The projects reviewed point to a number of nutrition and health components that seem to work well, but the project experience would not support a dogmatic statement that any given component or combination of components works best under all circumstances. It seems fairly clear, in fact, that no overall judgment concerning the inherent desirability of nutrition relative to health interventions is possible on the basis of the projects reviewed. The most effective projects seem to have featured a judicious mix of both nutrition and health components—a mix that has differed from place to place in response to dramatic differences in epidemiological, social, economic, and political conditions.

The experience gained from the ten projects also suggests that the mix will need to be varied according to the relative importance attached to different aspects of program performance. The Narangwal findings, for example, hint that nutrition interventions may be more effective in stimulating physical growth and reducing mortality at very early ages (particularly through maternal nutrition programs), while medical interventions may in general be equally or more effective, and also more efficient, in reducing mortality among older children. Under such circumstances, the relative importance accorded each component would depend on the priority attached to preventing the deaths of newborn babies relative to saving the lives of, say, toddlers two to three years of age.

The Narangwal data also suggest that more neonatal deaths can be averted than deaths at later ages for any given amount of money. This—coupled with the possibility that averting deaths at younger ages could have the further effect of promoting the kind of climate necessary for full parental commitment to the child, which could in turn help improve the child's physical and mental well-being throughout the critical early years and beyond—could argue in favor of placing greater reliance on nutrition programs that could be of special benefit to the newborn. There are, however, valid arguments to be made against such an emphasis. For example, toddlers might well be considered more "valuable" by both parents and economists in light of the considerable psychological and economic resources already invested in them.

Another dimension of the same issue concerns the importance that should be attached to mortality reduction relative to growth enhancement. It might be argued, for example, that a lower priority should be given to mortality reduction efforts than to program components that promote physical growth—in line with an overall policy emphasizing the capacities and qualities rather than the quantities of people who constitute society. To the degree that the Narangwal findings are more widely relevent, any policy decision of this nature would increase the importance of nutrition relative to health inputs.

These are difficult questions. The absence of easy answers, coupled with the situational differences noted earlier, argues against unduly strenuous efforts to "fine tune" intervention programs by identifying certain components as undeniably the most effective ones. Better to go toward the community with an open mind, and to be guided by the situation, the problems, the constraints, and the aspirations that are found upon arrival.

General Characteristics

From a consideration of the ten projects together emerge two other, more general characteristics that influence the projects' overall impact on infant and child mortality. The first concerns the degree to which the individual projects departed from the mold of Western physician-administered and institution-based medicine; the second has to do with the unusual effectiveness with which the projects' service programs were organized, administered, and directed.

Emphasis on Village-Based, Non-Physician Approaches. A principal characteristic that seemed to distinguish the more successful from the less obviously successful projects was the degree to which they departed from the

Western tradition of hospital-based, high-technology medical services in the search for approaches more appropriate to village conditions.

Illustrative of this is the role of the physician in the projects reviewed. Competent physicians planned and directed all ten projects. Even in the most village-oriented of the projects, physicians also played important roles in identifying problems, developing program approaches, training and supervising field personnel, and treating complicated cases. But in general, the more obviously successful projects were notable for their efforts to reduce reliance on the services normally provided by highly trained physicians.

Several of the most successful projects, for example, featured the development of simple medical care programs operated by paramedical personnel. Others emphasized nutrition monitoring programs designed to help mothers recognize problems as they arose, thereby lessening the need for physician-provided curative care. Several of the projects also demonstrated approaches to data collection and evaluation requiring few highly trained health personnel.

In contrast, the Many Farms project, judged by its initiators not to have been nearly so successful, was a conscious effort to transplant the high technology of the American medical school into a traditional setting. The area of the Rural Guatemala I project in which medical care was offered also featured a full-time clinic with a physician in attendance. (The nutrition services provided in another area of the project without the involvement of a physician appeared to result in better physical growth among children and lower child mortality than was achieved elsewhere in the project, although for a variety of reasons that finding was too ambiguous to permit a definitive judgment.) In Etimesgut, half the project's total expenditure went to construct and operate a hospital staffed by medical specailists.[18] The difficulties encountered by such early projects stimulated a search for new modes less directly tied to the Western practice of hospital-based, physician-provided curative care—a quest for simpler approaches based more on a direct appreciation of village conditions and the more central (if still incomplete) incorporation of village concerns. The degree of departure from Western medical practice varied from project to project, to be sure. Some experiments stayed relatively close to it by using paramedical personnel to provide the same kinds of services usually available only from physicians. Others sought to move further away from this Western practice, focusing more directly on the development of programs based on local realities, community resources, and the participation of the people served. All these efforts, though, were clear attempts to move out of the hospital toward the

---

[18] It is important to note that these three projects were among the earliest ones to be instituted—in the 1950s, when our understanding of developing-country conditions and problems was even more limited than it is now. Although they perhaps accomplished less in terms of mortality reduction than some of the later projects, all three made important contributions. As indicated earlier, the limited success of Many Farms gave rise to the concept of a "technologic misfit" between Western concepts of medical care and nutrition and health realities in the Third World. Rural Guatemala I made profound contributions to our understanding of the critical role of nutrition in child health. Etimesgut was able to achieve a dramatic, almost fully compensatory fall in birth rates within a few years after the infant mortality rate began to fall. By guiding and challenging those who sought to do better, both the results achieved and the difficulties encountered in these three early projects contributed importantly to the progress subsequently recorded.

village. The evidence summarized here suggests that the move was one in the right direction.

Leadership and Organizational Effectiveness. One cannot help but be impressed—in reading the project literature, in speaking with project directors, in visiting project sites—with how well the projects were organized and run. Service personnel generally were carefully selected, effectively trained, well supervised and supported, given carefully developed and realisitc duties to perform in a population sufficiently small to make adequate performance of those duties possible. Drugs, supplies, transportation, personnel, and other support services were usually available when and where they were supposed to be. The clinics and meal centers were open according to established schedules, providing the services called for by the project outlines. A service ethic, often inspired by a dedicated (perhaps even charismatic) leadership, was evident.

Such impressions give rise to a strong sense that the particular components of the projects reviewed were but part of the explanation of the projects' apparent accomplishments—that at least equally important was the effectiveness with which the particular components selected, whatever they may have been, were administered and implemented. This can hardly be considered surprising. However effective tetanus immunization programs might be in theory, for example, they can work only where there is a pharmaceutical supply system capable of regularly delivering vaccine to the places where it is needed, at the times when it is needed. Whatever the conceptual merits of the village-based primary care approach, it can be expected to have a significant impact only if program leaders are capable of implementing it adequately—capable of mobilizing communities; of recruiting the right people; of training, motivating, and supporting them effectively.

The project experiences indicate, in brief, that a health and nutrition program's overall effectiveness is likely to depend not just on what is done, but also on how well it is done. The need is not just for an appropriate mix of program components, but for an appropriate mix of *effectively administered* program components.

the need for caution in interpreting the results

Field studies are rarely flawless, and the ten described here are no exceptions to that generalization. The results of the projects should therefore be examined with a number of caveats in mind.

Problems of Evaluation

Village health realities are messy, and so are the findings of those who have tried to study them. As noted at the outset, the quality of field research in the areas of nutrition and health often has been inadequate for the kinds of analyses that would provide significant guidance for project planners. Although the findings of the projects described above are methodologically by far the best that exist and thus provide considerable insight into the efficacy of health and nutrition interventions and their specific program components, the data suffer from shortcomings that are significant enough to require mention.

First, the sample sizes in several cases (such as Jamkhed, Many Farms, and Rural Guatemala I) were not large enough for some of the most important findings to be statistically significant. This resulted occasionally from an apparent lack of understanding of basic statistical principles. Usually, however, the source of the difficulty lay deeper: study designs developed primarily to explore other issues proved inadequate for the examination of mortality change, especially when the relationships involved turned out to be much more complex than originally anticipated. The investigators who designed the Rural Guatemala I project, for example, were primarily interested not in mortality but in nutritional status and morbidity. They recognized in advance that the design they adopted, while suitable for their principal interests, was not fully adequate for mortality measurement. Similarly, the Rural Guatemala II study was intended principally to explore the relationship between malnutrition and child development, rather than between nutritional improvement and mortality change. The apparent impact of maternal nutrition on infant mortality through increased birth weights was not an expected finding. When it emerged, the study design, well suited though it was for the intended objectives, did not permit a fully satisfactory validation of this relationship because of insufficient data on infant deaths. Other projects encountered comparable difficulties.

Second, formal controls were often lacking (as in Many Farms, Etimesgut, Rural Guatemala II, and Hanover). Controls are particularly important for studies of infant and child mortality rates because the trends in these rates have been generally downward almost everywhere in the developing world since World War II. Thus, a simple decline in mortality rates is not enough to indicate that an intervention project was successful. Rather, the decline must be demonstrably *faster* than that occurring naturally elsewhere. This is very difficult to prove in the absence of a control group. To some extent, the shortcoming can be ameliorated by comparing project figures to national figures; but the almost inevitable existence of large inter-regional differences within countries renders this approach less than satisfactory.

Third, even when formal control areas were established, their populations and those of the experimental areas inevitably differed to at least some degree in ways that could have influenced the results. The Imesi project, for example, was undertaken as a service project, without a pre-established evaluation design. The control village, selected later, was probably as similar to Imesi as any other village in the area, but there were still important differences between the two. The same problem emerged in other projects, even when greater initial care was taken with the study design. The project investigators at Narangwal and Rural Guatemala I, for example, worked hard to find comparable areas. But their success was only partial: the areas at Narangwal had significantly different caste compositions, with all of the attendant implications of differences in customs and relationships within the community; the experimental and control villages of Rural Guatemala I had notably different earlier trends in infant mortality.

Another source of potential differences between treatment and control areas arose when, as was the case in Kavar and Jamkhed, the cooperativeness of local leaders was an important criterion in selecting the villages to be studied. Villages which in effect nominated themselves in this way could well have differed in important mortality-relevant characteristics from the more nearly randomly sampled villages that served as controls.

The experience of these projects suggests that, more often than not, villages in developing countries differ from one another in ways that are potentially important for infant and child mortality but that are not evident to even the most astute observers until they have actually been on the scene for a year, two years, or more. Some of these differences can be partly controlled for by statistical means. But this requires considerably larger samples than have hitherto been the norm; and, even then, use of such controls seldom leads to fully convincing results.

Fourth, the role of the interventions in bringing about the change in recorded nutritional status or mortality level was rarely established clearly and directly. Coupled with the problem of establishing adequate controls, this lacuna leaves room for considerable uncertainty about the importance of the intervention effort relative to the numerous other factors that could have been at play.

The Northern Peru project, for example, found large, statistically significant *infant* mortality declines in the villages receiving regular food supplements in comparison with the villages where no supplements were distributed. Yet the difference in the rate of decrease in *child* mortality was much smaller, and physical growth was not significantly more rapid among children in the villages receiving supplements. At first glance, these findings appear inconsistent. Perhaps they are not really surprising, given our growing awareness of the importance of maternal nutrition to infant survival, but the evidence necessary to determine whether improvements in maternal nutrition can in fact explain what happened in Northern Peru was not collected. It thus becomes difficult to dismiss the possibility that factors other than the food supplements—perhaps unrecognized and uncontrolled-for differences between the treatment and control villages—were responsible.

The same issue arises elsewhere. The Kavar project, for example, reported an average of 1.4 visits per person annually to a paramedical health attendant and modest improvements in domestic sanitation, such as the removal of household animals from living quarters, in about 30 per cent of the homes in the project area during its first fifteen months. The 50 per cent fall in the infant mortality rate seems extraordinarily large relative to the modest nature and volume of services provided. It may be possible to achieve so much with so little, but a further demonstration of a link between the services provided and the results attained would be very helpful in proving that unrecognized differences between the treatment and control areas were not responsible for a significant part of the results achieved. Similarly, further documentation of the contribution of the maternal care program at Narangwal would greatly increase confidence that the program was the principal factor in the large reduction of still births and perinatal infant deaths recorded there.

Finally (and as is usually the case when sophisticated statistical techniques are applied to large data sets), the factors that could be quantified by the project investigators—the program inputs themselves, plus other physiological, social, economic, and environmental factors—could not explain most of the total variance observed. About two thirds of the variance in weight among Narangwal children, for'example, remained unexplained even after program inputs, caste, sex, number of brothers and sisters, mother's age, season, and year of observation were taken into account. In the area covered by the Rural Guatemala II project, all factors together (diet supplements; initial maternal size, age, and parity; maternal home diets; and other variables) explained only about 20 per cent of the variance in child weight. Had similar analyses been undertaken in other project areas, they doubtless would have produced similar results.

Explaining even that much of the total variance is an impressive accomplishment, however, and many respected econometric studies have drawn policy conclusions from considerably less robust results. At the same time, though, it is clear that the projects' research programs did not come near picking up all of the factors affecting physical growth, birth weight, mortality, and other outcomes in the project areas. Had it been possible to identify and quantify these factors, the program impact could quite possibly have appeared considerably different (perhaps larger, perhaps smaller) than that reported on the basis of less complete analyses.

None of the sources of uncertainty discussed, of course, are unique to health and nutrition projects. Such difficulties, whether attributable to financial, time, or intellectual constraints—or to the limitations of even the most sophisticated statistical techniques—are inherent in field studies of this kind, no matter what the topic. The fact remains, however, that until such problems are resolved, the results reported by field projects like those reviewed must be interpreted with care.

Concerns about the Broader Aspects of
Interaction between Community and Project

Up to this point, our review has focused on the accomplishments of the projects with respect to the specific aspects of health and nutrition status that the investigators sought most directly to influence—particularly infant and child mortality and physical growth. But as the well-known WHO definition indicates, there is much more than this to good health—and good nutrition, which is so closely related to it; it is not merely the absence of disease or infirmity, but rather "a state of complete physical, mental, and social well-being." Thus, an appreciation of the projects' contributions to nutrition and health status, as more broadly and appropriately defined, requires an assessment not only of their efficacy in attaining immediate nutrition and health objectives but also on their impacts on many other aspects of village life—aspects which, while perhaps not commonly viewed as nutrition- or health-related, are likely to be of considerable significance to the development of long-term self-sustaining capacities to improve nutrition and health status. Two such areas are of particular concern.

First, none of the project investigators gave substantial thought to how their project might affect village productive and social structures.[19] Most of them were concerned principally with establishing working relationships with village leaders—simply to be able to do what they wanted to do in providing nutrition and health services. The few projects that tried to work more directly with poorer groups often met with determined opposition from village elites, suggesting the existence of sharp conflicts among groups within the villages and the importance that association with an outside group might assume in these conflicts. The Kavar project leaders, for example, quickly learned that they could implement only those aspects of the Chinese "barefoot doctor" concept that did not clash with Iran's strongly hierarchical village structure. As a result, they found themselves working through village leaders to a much greater degree than they had anticipated.

Other projects appear to have encountered the same sorts of problems; but aside from occasional passing references, the project literature seldom discusses the representativeness of the village leaders with whom the projects often, of necessity, became associated, or the implications of such association for overall village development. This gives rise to a concern that the nature and strength of village productive and social structures could well have been negatively affected by the presence of the projects—with especially serious consequences when village structures were characterized by substantial inequities in the distribution of power and productive resources. To the extent that village leaders became associated with or appeared to be responsible for the benefits

---

[19] Description of other projects that featured concern for this issue are to be found in the publications cited in footnote 8 above and in: John Briscoe, "Improving Health Care Where Health is Underdeveloped: Do Foreign Voluntary Agencies (Particularly Oxfam) Help in Bangladesh?" (Dacca: Oxfam, 1978); Zafarullah Chowdhury, "Organization, Supervision and Evaluation of Primary Health Care Workers," paper presented at the Ninth International Conference on Health Education, Ottawa, August 1976; and David Bradford Werner, "The Village Health Worker—Lackey or Liberator?" paper prepared for International Hospital Federation Congress Session on Health Auxiliaries and the Health Team, Tokyo, May 1977.

accruing from the project, the legitimacy of their position within village society and the existing structural relationships that they represented would have been enhanced. Since the inegalitarian nature of village relationships constitutes an obvious and important deterrent to overall rural development, and therefore to better health, even a modest strengthening of such existing structures could represent a significant loss for the society.

The complexity of these problems does not lend itself to a simple solution. Yet greater awareness of such issues and conscious efforts to deal with them are vital to the formulation and implementation of intervention programs. Too often the health and development literature calls for greater community partici- pation without a full appreciation of the serious difficulties posed by the redistri- bution of power and resources that community participation ultimately implies.

A second, corollary issue concerns the psychological impact of intervention programs led by outsiders. Although most of the projects subscribed to the idea of self-help, by and large they provided assistance principally from outside. Even the projects most dedicated to greater community involvement—such as those at Jamkhed and Kavar—found community mobilization considerably more difficult than the straightforward provision of services. To the extent that the development of a sense of self-determination is important to an individual's or a community's capacity to achieve better health, projects that fail to involve integrally the people they are designed to help may also diminish their ability to improve conditions on their own. Given the sense of dependence and lack of control over their own lives experienced by many of the rural poor—which may well have been generated or compounded by the inequitable structural forces mentioned above—there is a special need not only for sensitivity to the impact that projects may have on those structural forces but also for sensitivity to the perceptions of villagers about the extent to which they can participate meaningfully in the project.

No easy resolution of the potential conflict between the need for adminis- trative efficiency and the importance of seeing that entire populations are genu- inely involved in efforts which affect them so directly is readily apparent. Yet conscious efforts to reconcile them will be required if there is to be any meaning in the conventional rhetoric about the need for programs that go beyond simply helping people to helping people help themselves.

implications for future efforts

The Potential Contribution of Primary Care

The caveats discussed above are serious enough to lay to immediate rest any idea that the project approaches discussed here eliminate the need for long-term broader social and economic development trends to improve nutritional status and to reduce mortality levels. Far more needs to be known about the total effects of such projects, about their true mechanisms of action, and about their relevence for large-scale operations before their ultimate potential can be fully assessed. To claim too much too soon would risk diverting attention away from more general social and economic development efforts or from such other promising specific approaches as agricultural production patterns sensitive to local consumption needs and improvements in food distribution.

This having been said, though, the findings of these ten projects—especially the more recent of them—are obviously very encouraging. Taken together, they present a persuasive case that, in the hands of able leaders and in populations of up to 60,000-70,000, well-designed and effectively operated projects can reduce infant and child mortality rates by one third to one half or more within one to five years, at a cost of less than the equivalent of 2 per cent of per capita income—an amount no greater than that currently being allocated to health nationally.

Despite the many uncertainties that remain, results like these clearly merit much more than the usual glib conclusion "more research is needed." More operationally relevant research *is* needed, to be sure, and it should be pursued apace. But what is already known is more than sufficient to justify proceeding outward beyond carefully controlled field experiments like those described here.

This conclusion about the potential of primary care corresponds closely with the views of the many international nutrition and health professionals and developing-country governments already advocating the spread of primary care.[20] By doing so, it confirms that those urging greater reliance on community-based care appear to have identified a promising approach that deserves the further elaboration and refinement that can come only through experience with larger-scale service programs.

---

[20] Among the most noteworthy statements of such views is the "Declaration of Alma-Ata," adopted in the September 1978 WHO/UNICEF International Conference on Primary Health Care. World Health Organization, *Primary Health Care: Report on the International Conference on Primary Health Care, Alma-Ata, U.S.S.R., 6-12 September 1978* (Geneva: World Health Organization, 1978), pp. 2-6.

Realizing the Potential on a Larger Scale

Moving effectively from pilot projects to large-scale programs, however, is not likely to be easy.[21] The provision of services to millions rather than to thousands will require the development of management systems far more complex and more difficult to operate than those of the projects reviewed here. Also, the well-established health and nutrition organizations that normally assume primary responsibility for any expansion are far more rigid than were the small staffs that operated these projects; and at least some of those who lead and staff large-scale efforts will inevitably be less gifted, less well-trained, less highly motivated, less effectively supervised.

In view of the magnitude of these potential challenges, it is important that a review of field studies not limit itself simply to an expression of general support for the primary health and nutrition care movement, but that it also seek to provide as much guidance as possible concerning ways in which primary care might be most effectively spread. The projects reviewed give rise to numerous suggestions directed toward this end. Some of the suggestions are substantive, others procedural.

Substantive Suggestions. The substantive suggestions are straightforward, consisting of a summary of points made earlier. The contribution of nutrition to physical growth and mortality reduction in the projects reviewed, for example, argues strongly for incorporating nutritional considerations into program designs. Also, the transfer of health services from the hospital into the village emerges as a promising shift. More specifically, maternal nutrition and immunization, nutrition monitoring, and expanded roles for village health personnel seem to have worked well in many different settings. Yet, as noted, the composition of successful service packages has varied widely, suggesting that no single approach is best suited to all situations throughout the developing world. This indicates a need for considerable flexibility, a willingness to consider sympathetically a wide range of organizational and technological approaches developed on the basis of a full appreciation of local conditions. It is not enough for a proposed approach to be consistent with current international community thinking about what represents effectiveness; it is even more important that project implementors also demonstrate persuasively the congruence of their approaches with local realities, both technical and human.

---

[21] A possible illustration of the point is to be found in the initial published reports of the Bohol, Philippines project, which became available as this review was nearing completion. In Bohol, the infant and child mortality rates appeared to rise slightly during the project's initial two and one half years. The population served by the project was around 420,000—about twenty times the size of the population covered by the average project reviewed here. In addition, at Bohol, care was provided by the regular health services rather than by a team organized especially for the project. Whether these or other factors were primarily responsible for the difficulties encountered is not yet clear. The project is continuing, with special attention now being directed to the development of effective mortality reduction measures. (See Atkins, "The MCH/FP Approach," op. cit., especially pp. 201-2, for further detail.)

Another relevant study, which details difficulties encountered in moving from pilot projects to large-scale service programs, is David F. Pyle, "From Pilot Project to Operational Program: The Problems of Transition as Experienced in Project Poshak," Cambridge, Mass.: International Nutrition Program of the Massachusetts Institute of Technology, 1977, mimeographed.

Procedural Suggestions. The procedural suggestions result from the recognition emerging from the review that so many factors explaining the projects' accomplishments are very poorly understood, and that the projects may well have exerted unrecognized effects beyond those measured. The force with which considerations like these emerge from a review of field project experience leads to a strong sense that whether or not success is ultimately achieved is likely to be determined largely by how wisely and sensitively the field experiment experience is translated into larger-scale service activities. To be sure, the many distressing nutrition and health problems that now beset the world's children present a powerful case in favor of proceeding as rapidly as possible to expand and develop further the approaches whose trials have yielded such encouraging results. Yet the uncertainties that remain about the true causes and full effects of experimental accomplishments also provide a basis for concern about any transition from experiment to practice whose rapidity inhibits the reflection and continued refinement of techniques that will be needed if the promise of the primary care approach is to be realized.

Such considerations argue strongly for incorporating an introspective and developmental capacity into the primary care expansion effort now under way.[22] There is a pressing need for continuing experimentation and evaluation, with adequate mechanisms to assure that the results can be quickly utilized to improve service programs. There will be a continuing requirement for regular assessments of the extent to which large-scale programs are achieving the results expected of them, so that any need for "mid-course corrections" can be promptly identified and carried out.

These objectives might be achieved in many ways. Two particularly promising ones come immediately to mind.

The first would be further ongoing, larger-scale operational research and experimentation in the field, undertaken in support of expanding service programs. The ten projects reviewed here have demonstrated that results can be produced in small populations. The need now is for field research and experimentation focusing on the kinds of problems that will arise in programs serving large populations on a continuing basis. Ways will need to be developed, for example, to institutionalize not only the rules and regulations employed in successful small-scale projects but also the other factors contributing to their operational efficiency. Means will have to be found to reconcile the degree of centralized organization and leadership necessary for the implementation of large-scale efforts with the full local participation and responsibility that are essential to equitable programs. Experimentation is needed to find how primary nutrition and health care can be integrated with the more comprehensive basic needs programs that seem to offer the best context for nutrition and health care efforts.[23]

Field experimentation will also be needed for the development and testing of satisfactory solutions to the formidable problems posed by the vastly ex-

---

[22] The Alma-Ata Conference participants also recognized this need, to which conference resolution 16 was dedicated. WHO, *Primary Health Care,* op. cit., pp. 29-30.

[23] For a lucid presentation of the case for primary care programs executed in conjunction with other basic needs efforts, see James Kocher and Richard Cash, "Achieving Nutrition and Health Objectives Within a Basic Needs Framework," Cambridge, Mass., August 1978, mimeographed.

panded education and training needs of large-scale programs. For as the number of people required to staff programs changes from dozens to hundreds and thousands, field training will become increasingly important to provide the kind of direct, face-to-face, active learning experiences that proved valuable in the projects reviewed. Furthermore, as effective training and other program approaches emerge, continuing work in the field experimental areas where they were developed will become important for demonstrating to policy-level officials how the new approaches work.

Areas with populations of perhaps 100,000-500,000 would seem suitable for such purposes. In some cases, the experiments undertaken in them might be "test runs" of approaches under serious consideration for nationwide implementation; in others, where nationwide programs are already under way, the project sites could be used to experiment with alternate, improved approaches for later incorporation in the national effort. In either case, success would be defined not simply in terms of nutrition and health outcomes, but more broadly, to incorporate equity and community participation considerations.

A second, complementary way to help achieve the objective of effectively moving beyond the small project would be careful ongoing monitoring and evaluation of large-scale primary care service projects as they come into operation. The current prospect is that increasing numbers of large-scale primary health and nutrition care projects will be initiated during the years immediately ahead. As indicated, this development is to be welcomed. As also argued, though, overenthusiastic, unreflective implementation runs the danger of inflicting serious harm on a fragile, incompletely understood idea. This gives a particular urgency to evaluation efforts to monitor the progress of large-scale primary care programs and to provide early warning at the first signs of any failure of primary care approaches to live up to their potential. Only if such early indications of incipient trouble are promptly and unambiguously available can the necessary corrective action be taken before poor implementation damages the concept of primary care in the eyes of policy leaders.

What is needed is not sophisticated demographic research, but rather, simple program-management information systems that can be administered by program operators at all levels and that can provide them quickly with the information about their field operations which they need in order to assess their own effectiveness. Also important are the evaluation studies necessary to document the impact that large-scale, ongoing primary care programs are having on mortality—documentation that will be needed on that inevitable forthcoming day when policy leaders begin insisting on firm evidence that the funds they have allocated to primary care have actually produced the promised results.[24]

Closely related is the need—so essential but so widely ignored—for regular evaluation of program impact not only on nutritional status and mortality

---

[24] The primary care evaluation needed is, in a sense, the counterpart with respect to mortality of the extensive body of work developed over the past twenty years to assess the impact of family planning programs on fertility. Although family planning evaluation techniques are hardly without their flaws, they have been of considerable value in helping guide program development and in developing a strong case for the effectiveness of governmental family planning investments. This record suggests the utility of seeking to develop variants of these approaches capable of helping assess the impact of primary nutrition and health care on mortality.

levels, but also on the social and economic status of different groups. The ability of primary care programs to achieve good nutrition and good health can be meaningfully assessed only through evaluations of the broadest possible range of program impacts.

In closing, the initial question resurfaces: "Can health and nutrition interventions make a difference?" The evidence of the ten projects covered suggests a strongly affirmative response. Interventions are potentially capable of making a substantial difference. The need now is to translate that potential into reality.

appendixes
bibliography

.

Appendix A. Program Characteristics Covered by the Review

The following outline, which guided the review effort, lists the principal program characteristics relevant to the assessment of health and nutrition intervention projects; unfortunately, for many of the projects we reviewed, data were not available for all the characteristics listed here.

I. Description of the Intervention

A. Programmatic approach.
- Analysis of causal relationships underlying existing malnutrition, excess mortality, etc.; proposed mechanisms for modifying these relationships.
- General thrust and goals of program.
- Program auspices.

B. Population and setting.
- Where intervention took place, area covered.
- Size of total population in project area.
- Definition of the target population; size.
- Pertinent information on other demographic characteristics, geographic distribution of population, socioeconomic conditions, infrastructure, etc.

C. Personnel.
- Personnel structure and makeup; specific responsibilities at each level.
- If auxiliaries used: criteria for selection (gender, age, class-caste, education, etc.); whether local residents; whether full- or part-time; specifics of their training; interlevel personnel supervision and support structure.

D. Community involvement in analysis of existing health and nutrition problems; provision of personnel, clinic sites, materials; payment of fees, etc.

E. Detailed description of services provided, inputs; what services provided to whom, how often, where (in-home, clinic, etc.).
- Nutrition services: monitoring, supplementation, education, etc.; if food supplements were distributed, how much, to whom, consisted of what (percentage of daily protein and calorie standards), where and how often distributed, source of supplements.
- Medical services.
- Maternal and child health services.
- Environmental services.

F. Degree of integration of original intervention with local (traditional), state, or national health services.

II. Data Evaluation Framework

A. Basis for inclusion in intervention services: anthropometric status, at-risk models.

36

B. Data collection: longitudinal versus cross-sectional methods, etc.; if cross-sectional, controls for in-migration.

C. Control of confounding factors.
- Adequate comparison groups: how determined to be comparable, time series data, etc.
- Analysis for congruity using intermediate indicators.
- Stratification or control of expected confounding factors.

III. Results: Efficacy of Services and Programmatic Approach

A. Coverage of the intervention.
- Percentage of target population actually reached.
- Whether intervention (e.g., food supplements) reached target group in expected quantity; means of controlling intrafamilial food redistribution.
- Documentation of replacement effects.

B. Efficacy of auxiliary services: quality control, relations with the community, etc.

C. Effect of project on health-relevant community socioeconomic and political organization and on the population's capacity to participate in the solution of its health problems.

IV. Results: Nutrition and Health Outcome Data

A. Baseline and concurrent or post-intervention data on outcome variables for intervention and comparison groups.
- Nutritional status: anthropometric measurements, birth weights.
- Morbidity: respiratory and gastrointestinal infection rates.
- Mortality: neonatal, infant, young child, maternal.

B. Significance tests.

C. Hypothesized mechanisms for changes seen in outcome indicators.

V. Costs

A. Total cost of services provided (over and above health-nutrition services normally provided by the government, etc., in a similar non-intervention setting); cost of intervention per target group member.

B. Breakdown of costs by input; cost of individual inputs per target group member; start-up versus ongoing costs.

C. Who provided funds for what aspects of program: individuals, agencies, or organizations at the local, district, state, national, or international level.

VI. Replication

A. Replication attempts: auspices, scale, outcome data, ability to implement intervention on large scale with intent, characteristics, spirit intact.

B. Bureaucratic or administrative obstacles to large-scale implementation.

Appendix B. The Ten Projects in Brief: Individual Profiles

1. MANY FARMS, U.S.A.

In 1955, responsibility for the health of U.S. Indians was shifted from the Interior Department to the Department of Health, Education, and Welfare (HEW). To help develop an approach appropriate to American Indian conditions, HEW in that same year contracted with the Cornell University Medical School to organize a pilot health and medical care project among the Navajo Indians.

Cornell was a logical choice because its researchers had been working in the central Navajo reservation hospital for three years testing an antituberculosis drug developed at Cornell. The initial work had proven highly successful, and the Cornell team was eager to introduce the new drug more widely into the community, as well as to explore other ways in which modern medical technology might help improve Navajo health conditions.

Because the earlier experience had demonstrated that Navajo acceptance of Western medicine depended upon its compatability with traditional Navajo healing methods and religious beliefs, anthropologists were added to the project. It thus became an attempt not only to introduce new medical technology among the Navajo, but also to determine the extent to which an anthropological appreciation of traditional beliefs might enhance health program effectiveness.

The Setting

The Navajo constitute one of the larger American Indian tribes, numbering some 85,000 people living principally on their ancestral lands in northeastern Arizona. That land, now a reservation, is a remote, semi-arid plateau that receives 12 to 15 inches of rain annually. The population density at the time of the study was three to four people per square mile, with families living in widely dispersed homesteads. Per capita income was around $150 per year, compared with the U.S. average that was then about $2,500. Income came from raising sheep, weaving rugs, working silver, doing a little dryland farming, and undertaking unskilled railroad work off the reservation. Most of the reservation's roads were unpaved. Most dwelling units were windowless, dirt-floored hogans made of logs and mud. There were no latrines or running water; water was carried to homesteads from up to ten miles away. Most of the population spoke no English. The infant mortality rate was around 75 per 1,000 live births.

The study site, the Many Farms-Rough Rock community, was an area of 800 square miles located near the center of the Navajo reservation. It was inhabited by around 2,000 people whose living conditions were typical of those found throughout the area.

Services Provided

The project offered health care from 1956 until 1962. The package of services provided featured the standard curative procedures best known to U.S. medical schools. The project's headquarters was a new, well-equipped health center with two physicians and supporting personnel in attendance. Patients were usually given care at the health center but, when necessary, they were visited in their homes. People with complicated medical problems were transported to the reservation hospital 55 miles away, or to the government hospital 90 miles away. Immunizations were provided when appropriate but were not stressed. Nutritional considerations did not enter significantly into the project's planning or execution. The medical services provided were extremely popular, and about two thirds of the population sought care each year.

While the resident physicians were primarily responsible for the services provided, the project also included the development and deployment of a new category of personnel—"health visitors"—who were to serve as a bridge between the "modern" Western doctors and the traditional Navajo patients. The eight health visitors were all Navajos, four men and four women, with five to twelve years of general education. Most had been patients in the tuberculosis project and had an understanding of at least some health concepts. Their medical training by project staff members lasted four to six months, during which time they were taught basic facts about health and disease. Then, with the help of the project's anthropologists, they developed ways of explaining them to other Navajos. Selected nursing procedures, data collection methods, and first aid measures were also taught. The health visitors served as both clinic aides and as extension agents, performing relatively simple medical tasks at far-flung homesteads under the direction of physicians and nurses at the center, to whom they were linked by radio-telephone.

The Navajo tribal leaders were carefully involved in the project's execution from its beginning. The earlier Cornell tuberculosis work had been partly supported by two $10,000 grants to Cornell from the Navajo Tribal Council, and the Council was a joint sponsor with Cornell of the health care project. The Council helped select Many Farms as the project's site, the Cornell project leaders reported regularly to the Council, and project reports contain repeated references to the guidance provided by Council members on how to deal with local issues.

Evaluation Design

The project was not designed to permit a careful determination of its impact on infant and child mortality rates. All who embarked on the project were fully confident that the services offered would result in major health benefits if the people in need of service could be reached. There was thus less interest in measuring percisely the magnitude of the project's impact on death rates than in solving the formidable operational problems involved in the provision of modern medical services to a dispersed, traditional population. The principal research foci were clinical (tuberculosis and congenital hip disease) and anthropological (the cross-cultural aspects of health service delivery). The data necessary for such studies were collected from carefully maintained clinic records, from annual population censuses taken by the health visitors, and from special examinations of randomly selected members of the Many Farms population.

Research Findings

Table B-1 presents the limited mortality data available. Over the life of the project, the infant mortality rate fell from 115.8 per 1,000 live births in 1957 to 76.1 in 1961. The pace of decline was erratic; and during the project's last two years the infant mortality rate rose substantially. There was no control area; and within the project area the annual number of infant deaths was too small for the observed changes in the mortality rate to be statistically significant.

Table B-1. Many Farms, U.S.A.: Births, Infant Deaths, and Infant Mortality Rates, 1957-61

	1957	1958	1959	1960	1961
Number of Live Births	95	100	94	105	92
Number of Infant Deaths	11	7	2	7	7
Infant Mortality Rate (deaths per 1,000 live births)	115.8	70.0	21.3	66.7	76.1

The investigators reported notable progress against tuberculosis and against ear infections, neither of which was a major cause of death among the young. But the project had little impact on pneumonia and diarrhea, which together accounted for the largest number of infant deaths. The investigators concluded that their approach had failed to affect infant mortality significantly because of the inability of the modern medical approach employed to influence the diarrhea-pneumonia complex.

No data on child mortality or on infant and child growth were collected.

Costs

No cost information was presented. The maintenance of two full-time physicians as well as supporting personnel to serve a population of 2,000 suggests a relatively high per capita cost compared to that of the other projects reviewed.

2. RURAL GUATEMALA I

The first of the two large, extended nutrition and health intervention field studies thus far conducted by the Nutrition Institute of Central America and Panama (known by its Spanish acronym INCAP) was designed to explore the relationship between infection and nutritional status. The clinical literature was pointing increasingly toward a synergistic relationship between them; field work was necessary to find out how significant the relationship actually was in the developing world.

Achievement of this research objective in rural Guatemala required an intervention rather than a strictly observational approach. Virtually all children in the region were seriously malnourished. Only by supplementing the diets of some could the investigators obtain a group of relatively well-nourished children for the purpose of determining whether good nutritional status is associated with a lower incidence of infection. An intervention strategy was thus adopted in order primarily to facilitate an assessment of the basic relationship between infection and nutrition, and only secondarily to test the efficacy of the particular intervention approach selected.

The Setting

The study was conducted from 1959 to 1964 in three villages in the highlands of Guatemala, 25 to 50 kilometers west of Guatemala City. The villages were 10 to

40

20 kilometers from one another, with little communication among them. The total population of the three villages was about 3,000. The principal economic activity in all three was agriculture, supplemented by home weaving. The population was principally of the Mayan Indian stock that is predominant in the area.

From 30 to 60 per cent of the population, depending on the village, lived in thatched huts (rather than in more solid brick or adobe, tile-roofed houses). From 20 to 100 per cent lived more than two hundred meters from a public water source. At the outset of the study, from 40 to 70 per cent of the infants suffered from one or more intestinal parasites. From 30 to 50 per cent were significantly malnourished (i.e., 25 per cent or more were below the U.S. weight-for-age standard), and infant mortality rates ranged from 136 to 186 per 1,000 live births, compared with the reported national average of 120.

Services Provided

One of the three villages was provided only with nutrition services, consisting of supplementary feeding and nutrition education. All children under five were offered a daily food supplement that provided 100 per cent of the average child's protein need, and one third of the average child's calorie requirement. The supplement was available at a central distribution center six days a week. Daily supplements were also taken to the homes of pregnant women, nursing mothers, and sick children. Simultaneously, INCAP staff members instructed influential village women in good nutritional practices, and these women in turn provided instruction to others in the village. Nutrition education was also given during fortnightly home visits by the project's village health workers.

About half the village's children participated regularly in the food supplement program during the project's first year, receiving 75 per cent or more of the food supplement offered. This proportion declined steadily—to one third in the study's fourth year and one fifth in its final year.

The second experimental village received only health services, curative and preventive, designed to reduce infection without directly affecting nutritional status. The service program had five principal components: a medical clinic with a full-time physician and a full-time public health nurse, the creation of a safe and continuous water supply, assistance in the construction and use of sanitary household privies, immunizations against common childhood infections, and the efforts of a full-time sanitarian to promote better hygienic practices.

Acceptance of the clinic was immediate, and its popularity remained high throughout the duration of the study. Every village child was treated for illness at least once, and most of the children visited the clinic several times during the life of the project. About one half of the children were immunized. Latrines were constructed but not used. The quality of the water coming from village standpipes was improved, and the amount of it available was increased; but increases in the use of improved water by the villagers were modest.

The third village served as a control. Neither health nor nutrition services were offered. In order to elicit the cooperation necessary for data collection, project personnel sponsored a variety of activities that, while popular, were thought not likely to affect the nutrition and health of the village. Movies were shown, athletic events were organized, schoolrooms were improved, and the three-kilometer trail to the nearest highway was improved. In a few instances, emergency medical care dictated by ethical considerations was provided.

In none of the three villages did the project incorporate efforts to train and deploy new types of paramedical personnel. Nor was there any systematic attempt to involve community leaders centrally in program design and implementation.

Evaluation Design

The significance of differing infection loads and nutritional states was to be assessed by comparing the incidence of illness and the physical growth of children from birth to the age of five in the three villages during the period of the study. Measurement of the impact of health and nutrition services on infant and child mortality rates was a secondary rather than a primary objective, since the study's designers were aware that the number of deaths would probably be too small to support statistically significant conclusions.

Data on illnesses and deaths among children were collected by resident lay investigators, two in each village, whose six to twelve years of education had been supplemented by special INCAP training. They visited each home every fifteen days. In addition, each child was given a quarterly physical examination that included the anthropometric measurements that served as the principal indices of nutritional status. Annual censuses provided information on household size, composition, and socioeconomic status. Dietary surveys were also undertaken annually.

Research Findings

Growth. There was no significant difference in the growth rates of children in the control village relative to those of children in the village receiving medical care, but children in the village receiving nutrition services grew more rapidly after about twelve months of age. At five years, the typical nutrition village child weighed about one kilogram more than the 15-16 kilograms of the average child

Table B-2. Three Guatemalan Villages: Infant and Child Mortality Rates, 1950-59 and 1959-64

	Infant Deaths				
	Before Study, 1950-59		During Study, 1959-64		Per Cent Change
	per 1,000 live births	*(actual)*	*per 1,000 live births*	*(actual)*	
Health Care Village	136	(56)	88	(23)	− 35
Nutrition Care Village	182	(56)	146	(146)	− 21
Control Village	186	(115)	191	(70)	+ 3
	Child Deaths				
	Before Study, 1950-59		During Study, 1959-64 .		Per Cent Change
	per 1,000 children 1-5 years	*(actual)*	*per 1,000 children 1-5 years*	*(actual)*	
Health Care Village	50	(46)	34.5	(25)	− 31
Nutrition Care Village	55.6	(40)	24.3	(11)	− 56
Control Village	81	(101)	50	(42)	− 38

in the medical care or control villages, and was about three centimeters, or 2 to 3 per cent, taller. The height and weight differences were large enough both to be significant statistically at the .01 level and, in the opinion of the investigators, to affect physical functioning. They were not, however, adequate to lessen significantly the large difference in size between Guatemalan children and U.S. children. Children in all three villages consumed about the same number of calories during the study period; but protein intakes were 20 to 30 per cent higher in the food supplement village, suggesting an association between the protein-rich food supplement and the more rapid growth observed.

Mortality. Table B-2 summarizes mortality trends in the three villages. The infant mortality rate fell notably in both treatment villages but rose slightly in the control village. The child mortality rate fell in all three villages, but somewhat more rapidly in the nutrition care village than in the health care and control villages.

Only in the nutrition care village did the trend of infant mortality during the experiment differ from that which had earlier prevailed. There, the fall recorded represented a distinct departure from the stable level of the previous decade. The decline in the health care village, on the other hand, was no faster than that observed before the experiment began; and the slight rise reported in the control village also represented a continuation of the past trend. The declines in child mortality were about 50 per cent more rapid than the past downward trend in the health care village, and three times more rapid in the nutrition care village. It was also much more rapid than expected in the control village, where there had been no change in the child mortality rate during the preceding decade. The findings in the health care village were rendered less certain than those of the other villages by two epidemics of infant and child diarrhea during the study period's five years.

Costs

According to the project reports, the nutrition and health care services provided were designed to be within the financial means of the villages served. No more specific cost information was available.

3. IMESI, NIGERIA

The Imesi project, an offshoot of the services provided since 1920 by a Methodist mission hospital (Wesley Guild Hospital) in the town of Ilesha, was a service-oriented effort. Beginning in the mid-1950s, the hospital established childcare clinics in eight nearby villages. The clinic in Imesi, one of the eight villages, was selected as the site of continuing studies of nutrition and health conditions, and of the effectiveness of intervention measures in ameliorating them. The project was marked by a special effort to develop services on the basis of the health and social conditions observed in Imesi, and, by so doing, to avoid using European and U.S. models as the starting points in designing intervention programs.

The Setting

Imesi, a village of 6,000 people, and Ilesha, a town with a population of between 100,000 and 150,000 about fifteen miles away, are located approximately 100 miles north of Lagos in the cocoa-growing region of western Nigeria. Both Imesi and Ilesha are inhabited by members of the large Yoruba tribe, which constitutes about one fifth of Nigeria's total population. When the study began, the area's relatively prosperous economy was predominantly agricultural, with both cash crops (principally cocoa) and food crops (rice, yams) being grown. Overall food availability was generally considered adequate, although subject to the protein limitations of a cassava- or yam-based diet. Malaria was prevalent in the area. As in other parts of sub-Sahara Africa, infant and child mortality rates were extremely high, the official infant mortality rate for Nigeria as a whole in the mid-1960s being about 180. The area's social and economic structures were relatively egalitarian, lacking the obvious extremes in status and wealth often seen elsewhere in the developing world.

Services Provided

The service program was based on a study of the health problems of some 400 infants born in 1957, which showed that the three leading health problems among infants and children were diarrhea, pneumonia, and malnutrition. Malaria, whooping cough, and measles were also found to be major causes of death.

The approach developed to handle this group of health problems featured a clinic staffed by paramedical personnel who offered diagnostic, preventive, and curative services for all children under five years of age. (Thus the well-known name, "under-fives clinic.") The clinic operated seven hours a day, six days a week, with clinic personnel (many of them Imesi residents) on call at all other times as well. Mothers were encouraged to bring both well and ill children to the clinic frequently for examination: once weekly up to three months of age, once monthly from three months to three years, and once every three months thereafter, plus such other visits as might be necessary for specific problems.

The first step in the regular physical examination procedure developed at Imesi was to weigh the infant or child. Weight and other information were recorded on a "road to health" card, kept by the mother, which was designed to permit an easy comparison of actual weight with desirable weight at different ages. A child's failure to achieve an adequate weight prompted vigorous nutrition education of the mother, with nutrition supplements provided as necessary. Clinic attendance provided an opportunity to administer such routine immunizations as smallpox, DPT (tripple antigen for diphtheria, whooping cough, and tetanus), and BCG for tuberculosis. Working from simple standing orders, the clinic's paramedical staff routinely administered antibiotics, anti-malarial drugs, and other medications without consulting a physician. The clinic also contained a maternity facility where midwives provided both antenatal and obstetrical care. Other adults as well as children over five were also treated upon request.

Few services were provided outside the clinic. In particularly serious cases, project personnel made house calls to attend to children's needs. But the project reports contain no references to environmental service efforts or to other community services.

The project proved extremely popular, and wide population coverage was achieved. By the mid-1960s, some eight or nine years after the project's initiation, more than 95 per cent of Imesi's children were visiting the clinic on an average of once every two weeks. Immunizations were being given to 80 to 90 per cent of the children, and 90 per cent of all deliveries were being handled at the clinic. The clinic was also attracting substantial numbers of infants and children from neighboring villages.

The investigators attributed the clinic's drawing power principally to its ability to serve children with minimum delay, which resulted in a significant cost saving in a society with economically active mothers, and to its ability (unusual by local standards) to keep drugs and other medical supplies regularly in stock and staff available at almost all times. (Outside evaluations of the project made a point of noting the central role of its gifted leadership in the achievement of such efficiency.)

The project did not seek to develop new categories of paramedical personnel. The emphasis, rather, was on increasing the amount of authority delegated to the nurses and midwives who already played important supporting roles in the Nigerian health structure. A physician was present at Imesi only once every week or two. Clinic services were supervised primarily by nurses (with ten to twelve years of general education and approximately three years of medical education). The principal service providers were midwives with about eight years of general education and two years of medical training. In all, the Imesi project employed two nurses and six midwives for a total population of about 6,000, of which about 1,200 were infants and children.

The clinic's relations with the community appear to have been excellent, although the project reports give no indication that representatives of the community were actually involved in project decisions. The people did participate financially, however: patient fees for maternity care and adult services, which amounted to 40 per cent of the project's revenue, were essential to its operation.

Evaluation Design

Because the Imesi project was primarily a service effort directed toward helping the people of the area rather than a scientific field experiment, research was a secondary activity. The project was undertaken without a rigid initial evaluation design. Efforts at evaluation came later and were of two types.

The first was an informal comparison of infant and child mortality rates in Imesi before and after the project's initiation. Undertaken by the project leadership, it was based on project data for the latter period and on mothers' memories for the former.

The second was a much more intensive comparison, by an outside investigator, of Imesi's nutrition, illness, and mortality conditions with those of a nearby village, Oke Mesi, with a population of approximately 3,500. Births and deaths were recorded in each village for a full year, anthropometric measures were taken, and physical and other examinations were administered in both villages at the beginning and at the end of the year-long study period.

Imesi and Oke Mesi were both Yoruba villages, located about six miles from one another by path, fifty miles from each other by road. Social and economic conditions in the two villages were about as similar as in any two villages in the area, but they were not identical. The prominence of different crops in the two villages (cocoa in Imesi, rice in Oke Mesi) was apparently associated with somewhat different village ecologies and living styles. Literacy, for example, was higher in Imesi than in Oke Mesi. Differences in health service availability were significant, but Oke Mesi was not completely without health facilities. Also, although Oke Mesi had no under-fives clinic, the average Oke Mesi child visited the under-fives clinics in neighboring villages about seven or eight times annually.

Research Findings

The first, less formal evaluation in Imesi alone reported an infant mortality rate of 295 per 1,000 live births in 1957, before the project's initiation. The investigators found that figure had fallen to 72 by 1962. The 1957 child mortality rate was given as 277 per 1,000 children between one and five years of age; the comparable 1962 figure was reported to be 43. The number of deaths was small (18 infant deaths and 31 child deaths in 1962), but the differences between 1957 and 1962 were still large enough to be statistically significant at the .01 level, assuming that the mortality figures reported were accurate. The evaluation did not cover child growth and development.

The careful 1966-67 comparison of Imesi and Oke Mesi found more rapid infant and child growth in Imesi. Mortality rates were also lower in Imesi than in Oke Mesi.

From six to twelve months of age onward, children in Imesi were 0.3 to 0.4 kilograms (4 to 6 per cent) heavier and 1.5 to 3.0 centimeters (2 to 3 per cent) taller than children in Oke Mesi, differences that are in general statistically significant at the .01 level or better. Of the Imesi children, 38 per cent were below 80 per cent of the standard weight for their age (on the basis of the Harvard standard), compared with 49 per cent of the Oke Mesi children.

Table B-3 summarizes the mortality findings for 1966-67. The infant mortality rate was 57.3 in Imesi, or about one third lower than the Oke Mesi rate of 91.4; the Imesi child mortality rate of 18.0 was approximately two thirds below the comparable Oke Mesi figure of 51.2. The difference in child mortality was statistically significant at the .001 level. Because of the small numbers of deaths, no statistical controls for the social and economic differences between Imesi and Oke Mesi could be applied.

Among the program components identified by anthropometric and medical examinations as being possibly associated with the lower child mortality rate in Imesi were:

—Malaria prophylaxsis. The prevalence of malaria, as measured by the spleen rate, was only 10.4 per cent in Imesi, compared with 41.5 per cent in Oke Mesi.

Table B-3. Imesi and Oke Mesi, Nigeria: Infant and Child Mortality Rates, 1966-67

	Imesi (Treatment Village)	Oke Mesi (Control Village)
Infant Mortality		
Number of Live Births Reported	262	361
Number of Infant Deaths Reported	15	33
Infant Mortality Rate (deaths per 1,000 live births)	57.3	91.4
Child Mortality		
Estimated Midyear Population of Children One to Five Years Old	887	1,015
Number of Deaths Reported Among Children One to Five Years Old	16	52
Child Mortality Rate (deaths per 1,000 children one to five years old)	18.0	51.2

—Supplementary feeding for particularly malnourished children. As noted above, toddler weights and heights were greater in Imesi than in Oke Mesi.

—Immunization. Well over 90 per cent of Imesi children were vaccinated against common communicable diseases, compared with 45 per cent in Oke Mesi.

Costs

The total cost of the project in 1966 was around $12,500. About 60 per cent of this went to cover staff costs. Some 30 per cent was for drugs and other supplies. Roughly three quarters of all services went to Imesi residents, yielding an average cost of $1.50 per Imesi resident (the equivalent of about 2 per cent of the average Nigerian's income at the time), or about $4.50 per Imesi infant and child, after adjusting for the maternity and other adult health services provided.

4. NORTHERN PERU

The investigators, physicians at Lima's British-American Hospital, had become increasingly aware of the importance of good nutrition for child health and physical development. The principal determinant of the quantity and quality of food received by the child, they believed, was the quantity and quality of the food available to the family as a whole. The newly developed high-protein food supplements then attracting widespread attention seemed to have the potential for augmenting families' food consumption much more efficiently than had previously been possible. So the investigators decided to try supplementing the food supplies of entire communities with these new foods in order to accelerate growth and to reduce mortality among infants and children.

The Setting

The study was carried out in four villages located on a large sugar plantation in Northern Peru. The approximately 3,500 inhabitants of the villages were predominantly plantation laborers who received part of their pay in cash, part in food. Employment conditions were similar in the four villages. The ethnic and age compositions of the four village populations were also similar. Infant and child weights were comparable in three of the villages (villages I through III), lower in the fourth village (village IV). The infant mortality rate, while thought to be considerably lower than in other areas, was still over 100 in each of the four study communities.

Services Provided

The project's principal emphasis was on the distribution of food. For six years, from 1962 through 1967, the people of villages III and IV were offered regular food supplements. The inhabitants of villages I and II received only minimal services (occasional medical assistance and, in village II, a feeding program for toddlers during the study's final two years).

The weekly food supplement consisted of 500 grams of noodles for each family member. When fully consumed, the supplement provided an average of 250 calories and 7.5 grams of protein daily per person in village III. In village IV, where the noodles were enriched with fish protein concentrate, the supplement provided 250 calories and 12.5 grams of protein per person per day.

The noodles, collected each week by a family member from a central distribution point in the village, were to be prepared in the home. Ninety-five to 98 per cent of the families accepted and consumed the full ration, which was provided at no cost. Estimates of total food consumption suggested that the supplements displaced other foods, notably cassava and sweet potato. The noodles provided were of a type traditionally fed to infants and children, but the proportion actually consumed by children is not known.

Except for the occasional medical assistance and the meal program in village II mentioned above, no other services were provided. There was no nutrition education, no nutrition surveillance. Nor were any health services, clinical or preventive, made available on a regular basis. The project made no use of new or different types of paramedical or other community personnel. No effort to solicit community participation in the program was reported beyond obtaining the necessary initial consent of management and labor union representatives.

Evaluation Design

The evaluation plan was based principally on a comparison of the mortality and physical growth records of infants and children in villages III and IV, whose inhabitants received the regular food supplements, with those of infants and children in villages I and II, where supplements were not regularly provided. Data were collected every six months through censuses and anthropometric measurements. Frequent unannounced visits were paid to households at meal times to monitor food consumption. Mortality data for the twelve years prior to the study were also available.

Research Findings

Growth. From six months through six years of age, children in villages II and IV appeared to grow somewhat faster than those in villages I and III. (Village IV, with initially underweight children, received the supplement with the largest amount of protein; village II was initially a control village, but a feeding program for children was introduced in the project's final two years.) This result, which the investigators recognized as only impressionistic, suggested a possible connection between high-protein food supplements and physical growth.

Table B-4. Northern Peru: Infant and Child Mortality Rates in Four Villages, 1962-67

	Villages I and II[a] (Control)	Villages III and IV[a] (Treatment)
Infant Mortality Rate (deaths per 1,000 live births)	134.5	48
Child Mortality Rate (deaths per 1,000 children one to five years old)	40	21.5

[a] Arithmetic averages.

48

Table B-5. Northern Peru: Infant and Child Mortality Rates in Four Villages, 1950-61 and 1962-67

	Villages I and II[a] (Control)		Villages III and IV[a] (Treatment)	
	1950-1961 (pre-study period)	1962-1967 (study period)	1950-1961 (pre-study period)	1962-1967 (study period)
Number of Infant Deaths (0-12 months) per 1,000 Total Population	7.15	6.75	6.00	2.25
Number of Child Deaths (1-5 years) per 1,000 Total Population	4.30	2.05	3.75	1.00

[a] Arithmetic averages.

NOTE: Mortality rates are expressed in terms of deaths per 1,000 total population, rather than in terms of deaths per 1,000 live births or per 1,000 population aged 12-60 months.

Mortality. Table B-4 summarizes the results. The number of deaths was not large (between 60 and 70 infant deaths in all four villages combined during the period 1962-67, for example); but the differences in infant mortality between individual treatment and control villages were large enough to be statistically significant at levels varying from .05 to .01, depending on the villages compared. Child mortality was also lower in the treatment villages; but given the small number of deaths involved, the decline was not statistically significant.

Table B-5 compares infant and child mortality rates during the study period with earlier mortality levels in the four villages. As the figures indicate, infant and child mortality both fell more rapidly in the treatment villages. The difference between the treatment and control villages with respect to the rate of infant mortality decline was large enough to be statistically significant, but the difference in the rate of child mortality change was not in light of the small number of deaths recorded.

Costs

No cost information was available.

5. ETIMESGUT, TURKEY

The decision to implement nationalized health services on a province-by-province basis was made by the Turkish government in 1961. The Etimesgut Rural Health District was established in 1965 under the joint administrative auspices of the Turkish Ministry of Health and Hacettepe University in Ankara. While the Ministry has covered expenditures for the District Office, for each of the Health Units in the district, and for all paramedical staff, Hacettepe University has provided hospital services and medical staff. The program's objectives are: to provide integrated health and family planning services in all areas of the district, to establish training facilities for paramedical personnel, and to conduct epidemiological research relevant to rural health services and administration.

Auxiliary nurse-midwives are the key personnel providing health and family planning services in the villages and towns of Etimesgut. The nurse-midwives are supported in their work by referral and supervisory teams, each consisting of a medical officer, two public health nurses, and a medical secretary. The major causes of ill health among the vulnerable under-five population in the area have been identified as the general inaccessibility of health care and inadequate child-care and feeding practices in the home; in these circumstances, the resident nurse-midwives, reinforced by the team and hospital services, are thought to provide the most appropriate health service approach. Through continuous contact with members of the community in which they reside, the nurse-midwives can encourage the adoption of family practices that are more compatible with infant and young child health; and with the proper training, they can make appropriate referrals to higher-level care as the need arises.

The Setting

Etimesgut District, located just to the west of the city of Ankara, in 1969 had a population of roughly 55,000—including about 11,000 women of child-bearing age. Etimesgut's 670 square miles of mountainous terrain contain 84 villages and two towns. The district is traversed by three major highways and one railroad line. Daily motorized transportation to Ankara is available in more than one half of the villages and towns, as is telephone service. In 1969, 52 per cent of the total population and 41 per cent of those over thirty-one years had completed primary education—the latter figure was then equal to the national average. While the two towns in Etimesgut had piped water systems, nearly half of the village water supplies were found to be contaminated.

Despite substantial industrialization in the district during the second half of the 1960s, 70 per cent of the population were still involved in agricultural production; of those, 29 per cent were landless laborers. Average annual per capita income during this period was $240 for farmers and between $120 and $200 for workers. High rates of urban migration reflected national trends.

Studies on nutrition, growth, and development conducted in the area have documented protein-calorie malnutrition prevalence rates of between 15 and 29 per cent among preschoolers. The malnutrition-diarrhea-pneumonia complex was found to be the leading cause of death among infants and young children.

Services and Personnel

The Etimesgut Rural Health District comprises a district health office responsible for overall health planning and ongoing training of the professional staff; a

50-bed hospital, which operates in conjunction with the Hacettepe Medical Center to provide a full range of modern curative services; seven health units, each staffed with a referral and supervisory team as described above, and three to five auxiliary nurse-midwives; and 31 health stations. Each team staffing a health unit serves less than 10,000 people, with each nurse-midwife responsible for between 1,100 (in the countryside) and 3,700 (in towns) people. All team members visit communities and households on a fixed schedule. District residents receive free all health-team services, hospital care (if referred by the team), life-saving drugs, immunizations, and preventive health and family planning services.

At the program's initiation in 1966, public health nurses registered all families. The auxiliary nurse-midwives are responsible for reporting all vital events and migrations. They also keep records of their own activities and gather follow-up information on each pregnancy and birth. Twice yearly, public health nurses visit all households to verify figures collected by the nurse-midwives. Both the medical officer and the district health officer make spot checks to verify data collected on visits to unit stations and villages.

As head of the health unit team, the medical officer receives patients referred by the nurse-midwives, refers patients to the district hospital when necessary, supervises all preventive and family planning activities, and acts as a community health educator and development promoter.

The public health nurses have had four years of professional training after high school. Female nurses are responsible for in-service training and supervision of the auxiliary nurse-midwives, group education of mothers in child care and family planning, and provision of BCG vaccinations. Male nurses are responsible for rural sanitation measures, school and male adult health education programs, communicable disease control, and the twice yearly household census.

Auxiliary nurse-midwives receive three years of professional training after primary school. Seen as the most important members of the team, the nurse-midwives integrate the provision of maternal and child health care (including delivery supervision and scheduled immunizations) with family planning activities through continuous in-home visits. During home visits they identify new pregnancies and give periodic, scheduled examinations after the fourth month of pregnancy. Responsible for supervising home births, they refer high risk pregnancies to the medical officer or district hospital. Instructions on delivery procedures are given to parents when it appears that the nurse-midwife will not be able to attend a home birth. Frequent scheduled home visits are made for each child from birth to six years. Child care, nutrition, and family planning are discussed. Children are given tuberculosis, whooping cough, and tetanus toxoid (pregnant women receive these as well), and polio, smallpox, and typhoid vaccinations. Between 51 per cent and 88 per cent of the children aged one to four were given the various immunizations in 1973. The growth and development of infants and young children is monitored through measurement of height and weight; those with growth retardation are referred to the medical officer (details on the frequency of measurement, definition of growth retardation, and treatment or advice given is not currently available). Auxiliary nurse-midwives serving rural areas reside in the health station in the central village of their area.

Reported Results

Table B-6 presents neonatal and infant mortality rates in Etimesgut from 1967 to 1977 obtained from the household censuses taken by the public health nurses and for Ankara and Turkey when available. Infant mortality in Etimesgut

**Table B-6. Etimesgut, Turkey: Neonatal and Infant
Mortality Rates, 1967-77**

| Year | Etimesgut | | Turkey | Ankara |
	Neonatal Mortality (0-30 days)	Infant Mortality (1 mo.-1 yr.)	Infant Mortality	Infant Mortality
		(deaths per 1,000 live births)		
1967	36.0	142.0	153.0	101.0
1968	39.3	121.0		
1969	28.5	111.0		
1970	25.7	103.2		
1971	32.5	87.6		
1972	30.2	112.0		
1973	34.3	93.1	110.0	
1974	31.7	94.5		
1975				
1976	30.0	82.5		
1977	26.7	71.8		

declined by one third between 1967 and 1974, from a rate of 142 per 1,000 live births to 94.5. Neonatal mortality declined by 12 per cent in the same period, although there was considerable fluctuation. Despite its proximity to Ankara, Etimesgut's infant mortality rate in 1967 was considerably higher (142) than Ankara's (101)—although it reasonably approximated the Turkish national average of 153. By 1973, the Turkish national and Etimesgut rates had fallen to 110 and 93.5, respectively. Clearly both rates were declining significantly during the period, although the decline was somewhat faster in Etimesgut. However, without data from an area socioeconomically comparable to Etimesgut, it remains unclear whether the rural health program was responsible for the faster decline in infant mortality.

Costs

Initial investments and ongoing costs have been shared by the Turkish Ministry of Health and Hacettepe University, with UNICEF responsible for initial donations of motor vehicles, one X-ray unit, and other medical equipment. Hacettepe University finances some 60 per cent of total expenditures, including all hospital costs, while the ministry covers health unit and district office costs. Table B-7 presents total and per capita expenditures of the hospital and the health units of Etimesgut. Per capita health unit expenditures rose from $2.83 in 1968 to $3.17 in 1972, largely due to increases in staff salaries.

In 1973, health services in Turkey had been nationalized in 25 out of 67 provinces, with Etimesgut the only district where the model initially developed had been fully implemented, both in terms of sufficient staffing and of adequate training and supervisory activities. An estimated $185 million initially, and $100 million annually (or 2.4 per cent of the Turkish national budget) would have been required to replicate the Etimesgut model in all districts of Turkey in 1972.

Table B-7. Etimesgut: Total and Per Capita Health Unit and Hospital Expenditures, 1968-74 (excluding initial capital investments)

Year	Health Unit Expenditures		Hospital Expenditures	
	Total	Per Capita	Total	Per Capita
			(million	*(Turkish*
	(dollars)		*Turkish lira)*	*lira)*
1968	86,000		—	—
1969	93,300	2.83	1.4	27.70
1970	95,900		1.9	33.62
1971	173,300		2.8	46.78
1972	200,000	3.17	2.9	44.84
	(million Turkish lira)			
1973	2.3		3.7	57.00
1974	3.0		4.2	62.65

6. NARANGWAL, INDIA

The Narangwal nutrition and health project, active between 1968 and 1973, was designed to explore the effectiveness of nutrition and health interventions, especially the operational implications of the synergistic relationship between infection and malnutrition. Earlier research, primarily in the laboratory, had indicated that the combined effects of malnutrition and infection on the health of an individual suffering from both simultaneously were considerably greater than the sum of the effects of infection and malnutrition acting separately from one another. This was in line with, and contributed to, a growing realization that the diarrhea-pneumonia complex of disease, an increasingly important cause of death among young children in the developing world as specific infectious diseases were brought under control, resulted from the interaction of many factors rather than from any single, easily conquerable pathogen. It suggested by implication that the diarrhea-pneumonia complex might be treated most effectively not by medical or nutrition approaches alone but by a program incorporating both together. The Narangwal project was designed to assess the effectiveness of separate nutrition and health interventions, and to determine whether a combined approach did in fact work better. (A companion Narangwal population project explored the analogous issue of the effectiveness of alternative configurations of health and family planning services in lowering birth rates.)

The Setting

The project was undertaken by the Indian Council of Medical Research and the Johns Hopkins University School of Hygiene and Public Health in a rural agricultural area of Ludhiana District, in the state of Punjab, about 150 miles north-west of New Delhi. The population of the area consisted primarily of members of the Sikh religion (60 per cent of the study area population, compared with 2 per cent in India as a whole), most of whom were farmers. The study was carried out in ten villages with a total population of about 10,500, of which 1,000 were infants and children under three years of age who constituted the target population.

The study area lay in the heart of a region marked by rapid increases in agricultural productivity during the "green revolution" years of the late 1960s. This rapid agricultural progress had brought some improvements in health, but malnutrition and mortality rates among infants and children were still high. Although mortality rates among children between one and three years of age had fallen rapidly (from about 50 to around 25), the infant mortality rate had come down only slowly (from 155 to 130) and was no lower than the national average was then thought to be. Just under 50 per cent of the infants and children under five years of age (and over 80 per cent of the children between one and three years) were below 70 per cent of the Harvard weight-for-age standard.

Services and Personnel

Three forms of service were provided in the project's four study areas. One group of villages received only nutrition care—regular nutrition monitoring, se-lected food supplementation for children and pregnant women, and nutrition education. Underweight children identified through periodic surveys were served food supplements by project staff twice daily at village feeding centers (or, in some cases, at home). During regular home interviews, field workers emphasized to mothers the importance of late weaning and of consistent sup-plementation of breastfeeding starting four to six months after a child's birth. A second group of villages was offered only medical care. Field workers visited homes in the mornings, searching for and treating the minor ailments of children up to three years of age, and providing routine immunizations. In the after-noons, the field workers operated village clinics offering simple curative ser-vices. A physician visited each village clinic once a week and was on call for emergency cases at other times. Special features included emphasis on the use of oral fluids administered at home to treat diarrhea and of penicillin ad-ministered by paramedical personnel for the treatment of respiratory infections. Children and pregnant women in a third group of villages received combined care, featuring elements of both the nutrition and medical approaches, while a fourth group of villages, in which no significant services were regularly provided, constituted a control area.

In each of the three service areas, the primary providers of care were paramedical family health workers. Most were women with ten years of educa-tion, including two years of medical education. They were given six weeks of special training at the project, followed by weekly or fortnightly training ses-sions. Each of the twelve to fifteen family health workers employed at any one time was assigned responsibility—for both service provision and data collec-tion—for 65-75 children and their mothers in the combined care villages, 90-110 children in the other villages. They were able to reach almost all children fairly regularly, providing five to seven minutes of service on the average of once a week. Physicians, nutritionists, and public health nurses provided super-vision and support.

Community leaders were consulted regularly during the project's execu-tion, and community organizations provided support and assistance—buildings for village health and feeding centers, for example—and financial contributions to the continued operation of project-initiated day-care centers. Principal responsibility, however, rested with the project leaders who determined what service would be provided, recruited and supervised project personnel, and covered well over 90 per cent of project costs with funds raised from external sources.

Research Design and Findings

Evaluation Design. The 1,000 infants and children in the target population—and reproductive-age women, whose pregnancy histories were studied—were divided into four groups according to village of residence. Those living in the villages where no services were made available served as a control; infants and children in the villages where medical care, nutrition, and combined medical care and nutrition services were provided constituted the three experimental groups. The principal means of evaluation was a comparison of growth, morbidity, and mortality among the four groups between 1970 and 1973, a period that began after the services had been available for about two years.

Data for the comparisons were collected by the family health workers, who regularly recorded illnesses, physical growth, diets, and deaths among the children they served, following procedures designed by the project's research staff. The data were checked and supplemented by independent surveys conducted approximately once every two years.

Growth. Child growth rates were about the same in all four areas until children were approximately eighteen months old. Thereafter, it was significantly more rapid in the two areas with nutrition supplements than in the control area. Children in these areas tended to be 0.5-0.6 kilograms (6-7 per cent) heavier and 0.2-1.3 centimeters (0-2 per cent) taller than children in the control group at 36 months of age, a difference that is statistically significant at the .05 level.

There was little difference between child growth rates in the area in which nutrition supplements and medical services were both provided and those in the area in which only nutrition supplements were made available. Child growth was also greater in the area served by medical care only than in the control area, but the difference was not large enough to be statistically significant.

Mortality. Medical and nutrition services were also associated with significant declines in infant and child mortality; for some age groups in the service areas, mortality levels were on the order of one half those of the control area. As Table B-8 shows, the nature of the most effective intervention programs varied with age, nutrition appearing more important than medical care at the outset of life, declining in significance relative to medical care toward the latter part of the first year of life, and then re-emerging as a factor during the second and third years. The differences between the results found in the area served by the most effective intervention program and the control area were all statistically significant at levels varying from .05 to .005.

Costs

The most expensive of the service packages (nutrition care only) cost about $2.00 per inhabitant annually. The least expensive—medical care alone—cost under half that. Two dollars was somewhat more than 1 per cent of Punjab's per capita income, somewhat less than 2 per cent of India's per capita income, at the time of the project.

The cost of preventing a death varied with the age of the child, rising from

Table B-8. Narangwal, India: Stillbirth and Mortality Rates in Four Groups
of Villages, 1970-73

	Still-birth Rate	Perinatal Mortality Rate (0-7 days)	Neonatal Mortality Rate[a] (0-30 days)	Post-Neonatal Mortality Rate[a] (1 month-1 year)	Infant Mortality Rate (0-1 year)	Child Mortality Rate (1-3 years)
Control group	57	52	79	52	128	19
Villages with nutrition services only	25	37	48	48	97	11
Villages with medical care only	45	28	47	23	70	11
Villages with nutrition services and medical care	37	37	48	35	81	13

[a] Approximations.

$8-$14 for infants under one week of age to $31-$101 for children one to three years old. With respect to mortality reduction alone, nutrition interventions were generally more effective relative to cost up to one week after birth; medical care was more effective thereafter. Nutrition care was more efficient in promoting physical growth; health care more efficiently reduced morbidity.

7. RURAL GUATEMALA II

The second Guatemalan project of the Nutrition Institute of Central America and Panama (INCAP) was concerned primarily with assessing the impact of mild-to-moderate malnutrition on mental and physical development. Earlier research under carefully controlled conditions had given rise to a concern that serious malnutrition might cause significant mental retardation among children. The Rural Guatemala II project sought to determine the severity of the problem in the field and, in particular, to see if the mild-to-moderate malnutrition much more prevalent in the developing world were also associated with mental retardation after differences in intellectual stimulation received from the household environments had been taken into account. Operationally, the objective was to determine whether a nutrition supplement could help improve mental performance.

In the pursuit of this objective, numerous activities relevant to infant and child mortality were undertaken. The two most widely reported were the impact of food supplements given to pregnant women in increasing birth weights and thereby reducing infant mortality; and the influence of the project's medical services on infant and child mortality rates.

The Setting

The seven-year field effort, which began in 1969, was undertaken in four villages in the highlands of Guatemala, between 30 and 100 kilometers northeast of Guatemala City. The population of around 3,000 was principally *Ladino,* that is, of predominantly Spanish or Spanish-Indian culture. Subsistence agriculture was the principal economic activity in all four villages, and incomes were well below the Guatemalan average. Most houses were made of thatch and straw with dirt floors and occupied both by families and domestic animals. Average daily calorie intakes were also below the overall per capita calorie availability for the country as a whole. The infant mortality rate was on the order of 150 per 1,000 live births, some 50 per cent above the official figure of 85 to 90 for the entire country.

Services and Personnel

Nutrition supplements and medical services were offered in all four villages. The medical services were the same in all four, but the nature of the nutrition supplement varied.

In each village, nutrition supplements were made available to children up to seven years of age, and also to pregnant and lactating women. The supplementation centers were open twice a day, and all those eligible were free to take as much or as little of the supplement as they wished. In two villages, the supplement offered was a high-protein gruel ("atole"); in two, it was a protein-free drink ("fresco") containing about one third as many calories per cup as atole.

The medical services featured immunizations and ambulatory care, especially curative care, by carefully supervised paramedical personnel. Routine curative services provided by a medical auxiliary were available free of charge to all three mornings each week in a modestly stocked one-room clinic. Emergency assistance was given at any time. In addition, the auxiliary actively sought to immunize all children against measles, diphtheria, whooping cough, and tetanus, and referred undernourished children to the food supplement program. Beyond this, the program offered little health care or nutrition education. (It did not, for example, emphasize routine prenatal visits, delivery services, or well-baby clinics; nor did it include regular monitoring of nutritional status for other than data-collection purposes.) The average inhabitant visited the clinic about four times a year, and about 80 per cent of all preschool children were immunized.

The operation of the project's food supplement center was routinely handled by paraprofessional support staff. The auxiliaries who provided medical services had received six to twelve years of formal education (but normally no medical education). A brief (one- or two-week) introductory course covered the principal disease problems likely to be encountered and the standaradized approaches to be followed. The trainee was then sent out to the villages to work for three to six months under the direct supervision of an experienced auxiliary. Continuing intensive support and supervision were provided thereafter by a project physician who regularly reviewed all case records with the auxiliary, reexamined a sample of the patients to assess the adequacy of the auxiliary's work, and handled the 2-5 per cent of the patients that the auxiliary felt unqualified to treat.

The project did not seek active participation by the community. Staff members were selected and supervised by the project; all funding was from sources outside the community. The project's principal purpose was to test in the field scientific hypotheses developed by the research team rather than to provide the services best suited to, or most closely in line with, the desires of the people served. Arbitrary practices were controlled by the project leadership's insistence that staff adhere to carefully prescribed procedures, rather than by community control over the services offered. The project was not, however, totally divorced from the concerns of the people served. The original study design, for example, had called for food supplementation only, without medical services, but initial experience showed great community interest in and significant need for curative care. Thus a medical component was added.

Research Design and Findings

Evaluation Design. The evaluation plan was designed to examine the relationship between nutrient and calorie intakes and the mental and physical development of children, in line with the project's principal research interest. Different supplements were used in order to permit comparison of well-nourished, supplemented women and children with the less well-nourished women and children who did not accept the supplements. Comparisons were thus made among people within the different study villages, rather than between the entire population of the study villages on the one hand and control villages on the other.

Regular diet studies were taken to monitor the nutrient intakes of infants and children, as well as of other family members. A battery of anthropometric and psychological tests was developed and applied quarterly to determine physical and mental growth. Project reports indicate that birthweights, infant and child illnesses and deaths, and data about socioeconomic conditions were also recorded, but detailed information on the methods employed to collect these data was not available. Although no overall comprehensive report has yet become available, numerous research papers have presented data on child growth and development and on infant and child mortality.

Growth. Children between the ages of nine months and five years who regularly took the high-protein calorie supplement experienced gains in physical growth (height and weight) 10 to 15 per cent greater than other children, with differences statistically significant at the .05 to .01 levels. Children regularly attending the center offering the low-calorie, protein-free supplement grew no more rapidly than children not participating in either supplementation program.

Mortality. Prior to the program's initiation, the infant mortality rate recorded in the study area was 150, the child mortality rate was 28. In 1970-72, one to three years after the program's initiation, the reported average annual infant mortality rate was 55, the child mortality rate was 6. These latter figures represent a 60 per cent fall in infant mortality, a 75 per cent fall in child mortality. Infant mortality in Guatemala as a whole is thought to have declined during the same period by four points, from 89 to 85; and child mortality also by four points, from 26 to 22.

Preliminary exploration suggests that some 70 per cent of the decline was attributable to health care, about 30 per cent could be credited to the nutrition intervention. Tetanus innoculation for pregnant women was the most obvious single contributor by virtually eliminating the neonatal tetanus that had previously been a major cause of death. The most readily identifiable contribution of the nutrition intervention program involved the calorie supplements for pregnant women. Each 1,000 calories of food supplement consumed was associated with a three-to-five-gram increase in birthweight, after taking into account such factors as mother's home diet and mother's weight before the pregnancy. Five per cent of the babies born to women who had taken more than 20,000 supplementary calories during their pregnancies weighed under 2.5 kilograms, compared with about 20 per cent of the babies born to women consuming fewer than 20,000. The infant mortality rate was about 24 per 1,000 live births among babies born to women taking more than 20,000 supplementary calories, compared to 55 among the babies born to women taking fewer.

Costs

Cost figures for the program's nutrition component were not available. The health component was thought to have cost around $3.50 per capita annually, of which somewhat over one half was for medical supplies and most of the rest for personnel. This equaled about 0.5 per cent of the overall Guatemala per capita income.

8. JAMKHED, INDIA

The Comprehensive Rural Health Project, Jamkhed, Maharashtra, provides integrated curative and preventive nutrition and health services consistent with local needs and conditions. Community involvement in all aspects of the development and implementation of the project—from the determination of needs to the provision of services—is seen by the project founders as crucial to the long-term, self-sustaining development of health. It is hoped that the project, through its encouragement of analysis of needs, can be used to promote broader development activities as well. The specific goals of the project are to reduce high population growth rates and the high rates of morbidity and mortality among "under-fives," as well as to provide care for the chronically ill, particularly those with tuberculosis and leprosy.

Strongly committed to local involvement, the project directors first sought to identify communities sufficiently interested in participating in, and mobilizing their resources for, the comprehensive health project. The Jamkhed area of southeastern Maharashtra was chosen for its enthusiastic response to project objectives, as evidenced by the communities' donation of a site for the central clinic and willingness to provide manpower and other resources for the project. An advisory board, comprised of local residents representing a broad range of political and social backgrounds, provides liaison with both the community and government agencies.

The project, which began in January 1971, is still in operation as of December 1979.

The Setting

The town of Jamkhed, 400 kilometers southeast of Bombay, is located in Ahmednagar District, one of the poorest areas in Maharashtra. The project area, which originally encompassed a ten-mile radius from Jamkhed, had a population of about 85,000 in 1971. Initially, thirty of the local villages, with about 40,000 people, were to be included in the project. By 1976, the project had expanded to reach nearly double the number of villages and people, with a concomitant expansion in the clinic and field services available.

Agricultural production is the major means of livelihood in the area, with 66 per cent of the population cultivating their own land and 22 per cent being landless laborers. Although transportation in the area is poor, all project villages are accessible by dirt roads. Almost every village has a primary school, and the larger ones have secondary schools. Prior to the project's initiation, the area's health needs were being served by two physicians, ten auxiliary nurse-midwives, and eight basic health workers. Some eight to ten Aruyvedic practitioners were also serving the area's larger villages.

Studies undertaken before the project began indicated infant mortality rates ranging from around 80 per 1,000 live births in the town of Jamkhed to 150 in remote areas. Findings indicated that the malnutrition-diarrhea complex was often an at least related cause of death in infants and young children.

Services and Personnel

Efforts to meet project goals are being made through the establishment of under-fives' clinics emphasizing supplementary feeding programs, immunizations, and basic curative care; maternal and child health, family planning, and chronic disease programs; and a central clinic to make available to all surrounding villages more sophisticated medical care. Curative care is offered in part to encourage interest in the preventive and promotional health services offered, which are seen by project leaders to be of equal importance to meeting the project's objectives.

The project's special services for "under-fives" include nutritional supplementation (to "deserving" children) of one meal per day consisting of 50 grams cereals, 20 grams pulses, 10 grams coarse sugar, and 10 grams oil. Children under five are also offered primary care delivered at the village level, immunization (BCG, triple antigen, and polio), and semi-annual provision of Vitamin A to prevent blindness. Maternal health care services consist of prenatal and postnatal care for pregnant women, including tetanus immunization, and food, iron, and vitamin supplements; supervision of home birth; and referral of complicated pregnancies to the Jamkhed clinic. Other services offered include family planning, chronic illness control, blindness prevention activities, a full range of diagnostic and curative services provided by mobile health teams and at the thirty-bed clinic in Jamkhed when necessary, as well as public health activities, notably health education and environmental health control. Residents receive all non-preventive services on a fee-for-services basis. Services at the central clinic are available to all members of the Jamkhed area regardless of whether they reside in a project village.

Services are rendered by resident village health workers and by mobile teams of health professionals who alternate in providing care during village visits and at the Jamkhed clinic. The village health workers are local—usually middle-aged female volunteers selected from a group of three or four candidates chosen by the community to take on the part-time responsibilities of the position. At the outset of the project, these health workers received intensive training in maternal and child health and health education. In-service training provided at the Jamkhed clinic on two half-days per week includes group discussions, formal lectures, and demonstrations. Additional training is offered during the mobile team's visits to the village. The responsibilities of village health workers include the identification and follow-up of pregnancies; supervising home births; weighing and screening of under-fives for inadequate growth, diarrhea, fever, and skin and eye infections; supervising the supplementary feeding program carried out by other community volunteers (not all villages have such a program); collection of vital statistics; and the provision of simple primary care and health education to all villagers.

The two physicians who direct the project provide all of the training extended to both the village health workers and the mobile teams.

Changing village attitudes and habits detrimental to health is considered to be the most important role of the health workers. Because the health worker is a member of the community and therefore knowledgeable about its prevailing social, economic, and cultural conditions, she is thought to be best equipped—despite the rudimentary quality of the health care she is able to provide—to carry out the health, prevention, and educational activities. Moreover, adequate supervision and communication between project and village leaders can ensure that the health workers' activities are professionally adequate and meet local needs.

The mobile team that makes weekly visits to project villages consists of a physician, an auxiliary nurse-midwife, a social worker, and a paramedic—each of whom have had in-service training to help them carry out their specific duties within the village. Two mobile teams leave the Jamkhed center each day in the early morning, returning after visiting two villages each, one for intensive care and one for follow-up. The nurse-midwives are guided by "standing orders" outlining patient-care procedures, which enable them to treat nearly 80 per cent of all health problems seen; other patients are referred to the physician or brought back to the clinic, which has X-ray and operating facilities. When higher-level care is needed than is available at the clinic, referral is made to the Ahmednagar hospital. The nurse-midwife also supervises the village health workers' activities and provides follow-up on all pregnant women identified by them. Paramedics are primarily responsible for in-home identification of tuberculosis and leprosy. The social worker and physician also confer with community leaders on the project's progress and village needs.

Table B-9. Jamkhed, India: Comparison of Data in Project and Non-Project Areas, January 1971 and January 1976

| | Project Area | | Non-project Area |
	1971	1976	1976
Population surveyed	1,490	1,491	1,405
Immunization status of children under five	less than 1%	84%	15%
Infant mortality (deaths per 1,000 live births)	97	39	90
Antenatal care	less than 0.5% of all women	78% of pregnant women	2% of pregnant women

Reported Results

Table B-9 presents estimated infant mortality rates in Jamkhed at the time of the project's initiation and in January 1976. Comparison data from control villages are available for 1976 only. The decline in mortality in Jamkhed appears to be very substantial, as does the differential between project and non-project areas in 1976. However, without significance testing or information on data collection methods or on the socioeconomic comparability of these two areas, the efficacy of the Comprehensive Rural Health Project in Jamkhed in lowering mortality must be assessed with caution.

Costs

Start-up costs for the project—covering the financing of the Jamkhed clinic, staff housing, and motor vehicles—were met through institutional grants. The total annual cost of the program is roughly Rs. 400,000 (1978), of which an estimated three quarters is met by patient fees. The Indian government meets a small percentage of total expenditures with funding for specific aspects of the program, especially family planning. Annual per capita costs have been estimated to be in the range of $1.25-$1.50, or 1-1.25 per cent of annual per capita income.

9. HANOVER, JAMAICA

The design of the Hanover Young Child Nutrition Program resulted from the earlier experience of a rural health project (undertaken in Elderslie, Jamaica, in 1969), which had attempted to analyze local health problems and determine how to mobilize local resources toward effective solutions. The failure of the clinic-based medical services offered in the early stages of the Elderslie project led to the development of a community-oriented program implemented first in Elderslie itself and subsequently on a much larger scale in the whole of Hanover Parish. Hanover Parish, which comprises 177 square miles of north-western Jamaica, had a total population of approximately 60,000 and a target population (children 0-48 months) of around 6,500 in 1973.

The program began in eastern Hanover in 1973 and in western Hanover in 1974. Operated under the auspices of the Jamaican government, the project also involved the University of West Indies and Cornell University Medical College faculty and students.

Malnutrition was thought to play at least a contributing role in an estimated 60 to 80 per cent of deaths of children between the ages of one and four in Jamaica as a whole at the time of the project's initiation. An initial study of health conditions determined that infant and young child deaths constituted nearly one half of all deaths in the Elderslie area, with gastro-intestinal or lower-respiratory-tract infection often the most direct cause. Since curative medical care had been found to be ineffective in countering malnutrition under conditions of poverty and geographic isolation, the Young Child Nutrition Program was formulated with the idea fo providing modest, more appropriate services using community personnel and resources.

The development of the major service components of the project—anthropometric monitoring and in-home nutrition and hygiene education—was based on the conviction that resources adequate to the achievement of health existed within the community and only needed to be properly mobilized. It was thought that both the monitoring and educational activities could be used to promote choices concerning intrafamily food distribution and home food production that would be more favorable to infant and young child health.

Personnel and Services

Personnel. Services were offered primarily by 153 community health aides, with supervision, training, and support provided by an unspecified number of public health nurses as well as two faculty members and six medical students from Cornell. The community health aides' foremost responsibilities were anthropometric monitoring of all children under four years and in-home nutrition and hygiene education and demonstrations.

The aides received an initial eight-week training course in basic medical services, nutrition, hygiene, first aid, and family planning. Further instruction on obtaining census data, taking height and weight measurements, keeping records and plotting Gomez graphs, and teaching dietary improvements was provided by senior medical students. Continuing training sessions were conducted on a monthly basis in order to reinforce nutrition principles, home visit procedures, and program objectives. During these monthly sessions, problems and possible solutions were discussed with the public health nurses and medical students. No rigid protocols for the aides' home visits were developed in order to allow creative approaches to individual situations. The aides, most of whom were women, were community residents chosen from each electoral district by parish council members. The aide-to-population ratio was 1:391; the aide-to-target population ratio was 1:43, although an aide could be responsible for as many as eighty age-eligible children, because of variations in the accessibility and concentration of the target population.

In addition to training the community health aides, the medical students and eventually the public health nurses supervised the clinic activities of the aides, examined children found to be malnourished, and provided simple curative care.

Services. The program began in eastern Hanover in 1973, but was not implemented in western Hanover until 1974 due to a variety of resource constraints. A 1973 parishwide survey was undertaken to ensure each family's access to project services, and an attempt was made to identify all infants and children 0 to 48 months. During the survey, the program's purpose was explained to parents, who were encouraged to bring eligible children to the initial screening, which was held at a convenient location in each district. Weight, height, demographic and historical information was taken at the initial screening, and pre-marked Gomez weight/age graphs were plotted. Children considered to be moderately or severely malnourished (i.e., less than or equal to 75 per cent Harvard standard) became the treatment group. Field clinics were held at the same designated time and place each month, enabling continuing anthropometric monitoring and medical examinations of the malnourished. All other age-eligible children were asked to attend the clinics on a bimonthly basis for screening.

Dried skim milk, supplied as part of U.S. P.L. 480 assistance, was given to families of malnourished children at the clinic site in a two-pound monthly allotment when available; later, corn-soy milk was also distributed. Since these supplements were only sporadically available, and thus not thought by the project investigators to have a major impact on outcome, determinations of the amount received per child per month were not made.

Community health aides visited the families of malnourished children once or twice a week to discuss ways in which the children's diet could be improved by using locally available foods. The aides also demonstrated food-preparation techniques and discussed hygienic practices.

Evaluation Design and Reported Results

Data on the prevalence of protein-calorie malnutrition (PCM) were collected at the initial screening (in 1973 in eastern Hanover and in 1974 in western Hanover). PCM prevalence in 1975 was determined by a field survey employing the same methodology used during the initial screening. Data on PCM incidence were collected from monthly clinic records. Eighty-six per cent of those eligible in eastern Hanover and 97 per cent in western Hanover were initially screened. Lack of information on target population attendance rates thereafter and on procedures for following up no-shows and identifying new births and immigrants requires that these cross-sectional data be used with caution. Mortality data were available from records kept by local registrars and a local hospital. Death registration methods had not changed since 1971.

Table B-10. Hanover, Jamaica: Initial Prevalence of Malnutrition Among Children Aged 0-48 Months

| Gomez Grade | Eastern Hanover[a] | | Western Hanover[b] | |
	Number	Percentage	Number	Percentage
Normal	1,660	57.7	1,604	50.1
I	907	31.5	1,179	36.8
II	281	9.8	369	11.5
III	31	1.1	48	1.5

[a] July-August 1973.
[b] July-August 1974.

NOTE: Gomez grades are defined as follows: I, 75-90 per cent; II, 60-74 per cent; III, below 60 per cent standard weight for age.

Table B-11. Hanover, Jamaica: Prevalence of Malnutrition Among Children Aged 0-48 Months, 1973, 1974, 1975

	Eastern Hanover	Western Hanover
	(percentages)	
July 1973	10.9[a]	—
July 1974	5.9	13.0[a]
July 1975	6.2	6.6

[a]Date of program initiation.

NOTE: Malnutrition is defined as falling below 75 per cent of standard weight for age (Gomez grades II and III). The declines from 1973 to 1974 and 1975 in eastern Hanover, and those from 1974 to 1975 in western Hanover were statistically significant (p < .00005).

The sequential implementation of the program in eastern Hanover and then western Hanover provided the only control; there were no comparison groups per se. Time series mortality data were obtained from 1971 on—in order to verify the trend of slowly declining mortality prior to program implementation. The authors of the reported results assert that no discernible changes took place in socioeconomic conditions after the program began. Outside investigators, however, have pointed to the opening of the Cornwall Regional Hospital in nearby St. James Parish as possibly having significant impact on subsequent infant mortality rates in Hanover.

Nutritional Status. Table B-10 presents data on initial PCM prevalence in eastern and western Hanover. Table B-11 presents PCM prevalence data from both areas for 1973-75. The declines from 10.9 per cent in 1973 to 5.9 per cent in 1974 in eastern Hanover, and from 13.0 per cent in 1974 to 6.6 per cent in 1975 in western Hanover, were statistically significant (p < .00005). The project investigators suggest that because analysis of outcome data assumed the population to have remained constant (whereas the population in reality was increasing), the declines in PCM prevalence achieved over this period were even more dramatic than the statistics suggest. An even more substantial decline occurred in the severely malnourished group (< 60 per cent of the Harvard weight/age standard) in both eastern and western Hanover: from 1.1 per cent to 0.04 per cent, and from 1.5 per cent to 0.06 per cent, respectively. Incidence of PCM was apparently unchanged by the program.

Mortality. Table B-12 presents mortality rates for children aged 1 to 48 months for 1971-76. Two to three years before the program, mortality rates for the same group averaged 14.5 per 1,000. Within one year after the program began, mortality rates fell by more than one half. The infant mortality rate in Hanover fell from an average of 36 per 1,000 in 1970-73 (while there was considerable fluctuation in the rate during this period, it never fell below 26) to 10.6 in 1975; these rates compare very favorably with Jamaican national averages of 26.2 in 1973 and 23.2 in 1975. Neonatal mortality rates were largely unaffected, remaining at about 8 per 1,000 live births.

Ongoing anthropometric monitoring, early identification and referral of children in need of treatment, and in-home nutrition and hygiene education stressing better use of available resources are considered to be major factors in the dramatic declines in PCM prevalence and mortality rates. While curative care

65

**Table B-12. Hanover, Jamaica: Mortality Rates
for Children Aged 1-48 Months, 1971-76**

	Eastern Hanover (n = 3,357)		Western Hanover (n = 3,294)	
	Mortality Rate	(Actual Number of Deaths)	Mortality Rate	(Actual Number of Deaths)
July 1971-June 1972	13.7	(46)	12.7	(42)
July 1972-June 1973	15.4	(52)	17.6	(58)
July 1973-June 1974	5.6	(19)	13.3	(44)
July 1974-June 1975	7.4	(25)	5.7	(19)
July 1975-June 1976	5.6	(19)	5.7	(19)

NOTE: The difference between pre- and post-project years was significant ($p < .001$).

aspects of clinics probably greatly encouraged attendance, it was felt that because of the nature of the illnesses seen and the treatment provided, medical services did not have a notable impact. Food supplements were thought to play only a minor role, because of an unreliable supply throughout the program's implementation. This conviction was strengthened by the failure of the government's milk-distribution program over the preceding decade to have an impact on child mortality. It may be that the field clinics provided a much more efficient distribution system than the government program, but without information on the amounts of the supplements provided, the time intervals of their distribution, and their utilization within the family, the impact of the supplements is unclear.

10. KAVAR, IRAN

In 1972, the Department of Community Medicine, Pahlavi University, Shiraz, in cooperation with the local Health Corps Station, undertook the design and implementation of an ongoing pilot project to train and deploy resident village health workers to provide basic curative and preventive health care. The limited medical care ordinarily available in rural areas is provided by the national Health Corps Stations, whose staffs consist of recently graduated physicians serving for eighteen months in lieu of military service. It was the view of the project's founders that, as a result of the maldistribution and severe shortage of physicians in Iran and the lack of health manpower alternatives, a significant portion of Iran's rural population does not have access to adequate medical care. The project was established to test the efficacy of auxiliary health personnel within the constraints of a rural setting in Iran.

Setting and Personnel

The villages around the Kavar Health Corps Station, which had a total population of about 20,000, were chosen as the project site because of their proximity to Shiraz (55 kilometers to the southeast) and the relative accessibility of the Station to the villages (distance of village from Station ranges from 2 kilometers to 60 kilometers). Village leaders or Council members in 40 of the 55 local villages and towns in the Kavar area were contacted during the preliminary process of determining which villages should be included in the project; final decisions were based on more thorough investigation of the availability of literate villagers who could be trained as health workers and the potential for community cooperation and participation. Although efforts were made to promote community selection of candidate health workers in the villages chosen to participate, existing social and political structures made it difficult to identify individuals who would be widely accepted. Due to very low literacy rates and the restrictions on the personal freedom of women, fewer female candidates were found than had been hoped. Initially, sixteen health workers were selected, ranging in age from 15 to 45 years. Eleven were male; five were female. At the time they were chosen, the villages they came from and returned to had populations of between 150 and 1,500. Villages with health workers are interspersed with control villages judged to be similar on the basis of a variety of demographic, geographic, social, and economic variables.

In August 1973, the first six-month training course for village workers began. (Training was subsequently extended to nine months.) The objectives developed for the training of village health workers—based on the findings of a seventeen-month study of health problems in a rural area 50 kilometers north of Shiraz—call for reasonable proficiency in the following fields: diagnosis and treatment of selected medical problems and recognition of cases that should be referred to the Health Corps Station; maternal and child health care and family planning activities, especially the referral of new or complicated pregnancies; communicable disease control, including assistance in immunization campaigns; nutrition, especially diagnosing poor diet or growth and prescribing appropriate diets and vitamins; record-keeping on vital events, weights and heights of village children, drugs prescribed and dispensed, and individual patient histories; environmental control; and health education. Approximately half of the course is spent in theoretical training, half in practical field experience. No single disease, identification procedure, target group, or treatment is stressed. Rather, it is hoped that through clinic-based experience with physicians and midwives, and preventive activities in the field, the health workers will learn to deal with a broad range of health needs within the community.

The first group of trained village health workers began work—on a part-time basis—in March 1974. Two were assigned to communities other than their native villages because local disputes (apparently of a political nature) precluded their acceptance and effectiveness under these circumstances. Before the health workers officially began their work, project investigators met with village leaders to discuss project objectives and the importance of community cooperation. Since the beginning of program services, community leaders, members of the National Development Corps, and all interested parties have been invited to monthly meetings held in each village to discuss project progress with the village health worker and training director.

A review of program operation at the end of the first year revealed that, as a result of the emphasis given to it in their training, health workers preferred to provide curative care. Given the importance attached to preventive and promotional health activities in program objectives, efforts have since been made to upgrade training in those areas. In addition, a middle-level auxiliary position has been developed to provide, in addition to direct patient care, some training and supervision emphasizing preventive and promotional activities. These auxiliary workers had the additional qualifications of a high school diploma (compared with the six years of general education required for village health workers) and three years of specialized training (compared with the six to nine months of training given to village health workers). The middle-level auxiliaries first began work in the field in the fall of 1976.

By the end of the first year of operation, when the demand for services necessitated that their previously part-time positions become full-time, village health workers received a salary of $75 per month.

Services

Morning clinics for diagnostic, treatment, referral, and record-keeping activities are held in sites provided by each village. Depending on patient demand, the clinics generally remain open for two to five hours. Referral of patients needing higher-level care is made to the Health Corps Station, to a hospital in Shiraz, or to the Department of Community Medicine resident acting as field supervisor.

Afternoons are spent in follow-up and well-baby visits and community health activities. Personal hygiene, household sanitation, and nutrition and family planning are among the topics discussed during home visits. The health workers are also responsible for the identification and organization of projects that will promote community health, such as campaigns for immunization, construction of deep wells and water tanks, and separation of animals from household living quarters.

The health workers' activities are supervised by a variety of project staff. Clinical field supervisors visit weekly to review the recorded diagnosis and treatment of at least two patients. The training director and environmental health specialists make periodic visits in order to oversee and provide suggestions for public health activities. Efforts are made to give encouragement as well as supervision to the health workers, both publicly and privately. Continuing education is offered in weekly meetings at the Station, as well as in refresher courses.

Clinic visits are free to villagers unless drugs are dispensed—in which case a small fee is normally charged, in the hope of reducing dependence on and demand for drugs while promoting utilization of the more prevention-oriented services offered. (It is left up to the individual health worker to decide whether to dispense drugs to those who cannot pay the fee.) No fee is charged when referral to higher-level care is required.

Reported Results

In June 1975, the first house-to-house census was conducted in all project and control villages. It was undertaken during a major harvest, in the hope that the previous year's harvest would provide villagers with a reference point for determining vital events over the intervening year. Since then, data on vital events have been collected monthly in project villages and tri-monthly in control villages.

Table B-13 presents infant and fetal mortality rates obtained from the 1975 census. Table B-14 presents vital events data collected between March 1977 and March 1978. Despite the absence of baseline data, the comparability between project and control villages—determined on a variety of social, economic, and demographic variables (a few of which are summarized in Table B-15)—suggests, according to project investigators, that the substantial differ-

Table B-13. Kavar, Iran: Infant Mortality and Fetal Death Rates In Villages With and Without Health Workers, June 1974-June 1975

	Villages With Health Workers	Control Villages	Level of Significance
	(deaths per 1,000 live births)		
Infant Mortality Rate	64.3	127.7	p < .01
Fetal Death Rate[a]	36	79	p < .01

[a] In a census of this nature, it is not possible to distinguish true fetal deaths from deaths very soon after birth, even though persons were asked specifically whether the infant was dead at the time of expulsion or extraction. The fetal death rate is defined as fetal deaths divided by live births (x 1,000).

ences in 1975 infant and fetal mortality rates between project and control villages are indeed due to program impact. Differences in infant mortality in 1975 (64.7 per 1,000 live births versus 127.7) and 1977-78 (84 versus 138) are significant at the .01 and .05 levels, respectively. Project investigators surmise that the apparent increase in infant mortality in both project and control villages between 1975 and 1977 is due to undercounting in the first census rather than to real increases. Differences in fetal death rates in 1975 between project and control villages, 36 per 1,000 live births versus 79, are significant at the .02 level. Taken together, the mortality data presented in Table B-14 indicate that the significant difference in the crude death rate is due solely to differences in infant mortality rates, other ages being largely unaffected. It was disappointing to find that birthrates were the same in project and control villages in 1977-78 (Table B-14); however, it may be that fewer stillbirths in project villages are masking a decrease in numbers of pregnancies (while the actual numbers are not available, stillbirth rates were found to be substantially lower in project villages in 1977—significant at the .01 level).

Table B-14. Kavar, Iran: Infant Mortality, Death, Birth, and Infant Death Rates in Villages With Health Workers and Control Villages, March 1977-March 1978

	Villages With Health Workers	Control Villages	Significance of Difference
Infant Mortality Rate (per 1,000 live births)	84	138	p < .05
Crude Death Rate (per 1,000 population)	14	17	p < .05
Crude Birth Rate (per 1,000 population)	37	37	not significant

Table B-15. Kavar, Iran: Median Ages, Literacy Rates, and Dependency Ratios in Villages With Health Workers and Control Villages, 1975

	Villages With Health Workers	Control Villages
Median Age, Males	12.3 years	12.5 years
Median Age, Females	12.2 years	12.7 years
Literacy Rate, Males	28%	33%
Literacy Rate, Females	6%	7%
Dependency Ratio[a]	1,051	1,021

[a] Number of persons under 15 years and over 64 years for every 1,000 persons aged 15-64.

Costs

Estimates of total annual recurring costs made prior to the deployment of the middle-level auxiliaries suggest an annual per capita cost of $3.54. When investment and training costs are added in, this figure rises to $5.35.

Bibliography
Principal Publications Covering the Projects Reviewed

Many Farms, U.S.A.
Adair, John K., and Deuschle, Kurt W. *The People's Health: Medicine and Anthropology in a Navajo Community.* New York: Appleton-Century, Crofts, 1970.
McDermott, Walsh; Deuschle, Kurt W.; and Barnett, Clifford R. "Health Care Experiment at Many Farms." *Science* 175 (January 7, 1972): 23-31.

Rural Guatemala I
Scrimshaw, Nevin S.; Guzman, Miguel A.; and Gordon, John E. "Nutrition and Infection Field Study in Guatemalan Villages, 1959-1964: I. Study Plan and Experimental Design." *Archives of Environmental Health* 14 (May 1967): 657-63.
Scrimshaw, Nevin S.; Guzman, Miguel A.; Kevany, John J.; Ascoli, Werner; Bruch, Hans; and Gordon, John E. "Nutrition and Infection Field Study in Guatemalan Villages, 1959-1964: II. Field Reconnaissance, Administrative and Technical; Study Area; Population Characteristics; and Organization for Field Activities." *Archives of Environmental Health* 14 (June 1967): 787-801.
Scrimshaw, Nevin S.; Ascoli, Werner; Kevany, John J.; Flores, Marina; Iscaza, Susana J.; and Gordon, John E. "Nutrition and Infection Field Study in Guatemalan Villages, 1959-1964: III. Field Procedure, Collection of Data, and Methods of Measurement." *Archives of Environmental Health* 15 (July 1967): 7-15.
Ascoli, Werner; Guzman, Miguel A.; Scrimshaw, Nevin S.; and Gordon, John E. "Nutrition and Infection Field Study in Guatemalan Villages, 1959-1964: IV. Deaths of Infants and Preschool Children." *Archives of Environmental Health* 15 (October 1967): 439-49.
Scrimshaw, Nevin S.; Guzman, Miguel A.; Flores, Marina; and Gordon, John E. "Nutrition and Infection Field Study in Guatemalan Villages, 1959-1964: V. Disease Incidence Among Preschool Children Under Natural Village Conditions, with Improved Diet and with Medical and Public Health Services." *Archives of Environmental Health* 16 (February 1968): 223-34.
Gordon, John E.; Ascoli, Werner; Mata, Leonardo J.; Guzman, Miguel A.; and Scrimshaw, Nevin S. "Nutrition and Infection Field Study in Guatemalan Villages, 1959-1964: VI. Acute Diarrheal Disease and Nutritional Disorders in General Disease Incidence." *Archives of Environmental Health* 16 (March 1968): 424-37.
Guzman, Miguel A.; Scrimshaw, Nevin S.; Bruch, Hans A.; and Gordon, John E. "Nutrition and Infection Field Study in Guatemalan Villages, 1959-1964: VII. Physical Growth and Development of Preschool Children." *Archives of Environmental Health* 17 (July 1968): 107-18.
Behar, Moises; Scrimshaw, Nevin S.; Guzman, Miguel A.; and Gordon, John E. "Nutrition and Infection Field Study in Guatemalan Villages, 1959-1964: VIII. An Epidemiological Appraisal of Its Wisdom and Errors." *Archives of Environmental Health* 17 (November 1968): 814-27.

Scrimshaw, Nevin S.; Behar, Moises; Guzman, Miguel A.; and Gordon, John E. "Nutrition and Infection Field Study in Guatemalan Villages, 1959-1964: IX. An Evaluation of Medical, Social, and Public Health Benefits, with Suggestions for Future Field Study." *Archives of Environmental Health* 18 (January 1969): 51-62.

Imesi, Nigeria

Cunningham, Nicholas. "An Evaluation of an Auxiliary Based Child Health Service in Rural Nigeria." *Journal of the Society of Nigerian Health* 3 (1969): 21-25.
───────. "The Under Fives Clinic: What Difference Does It Make?" Ph.D. Dissertation, The Johns Hopkins University, June 1976.
Morley, David. "A Medical Service for Children Under Five Years of Age in West Africa." *Transactions of the Royal Society of Tropical Medicine and Hygiene* 57/1 (February 1963): 79-83.
───────. *Pediatric Priorities in the Developing World*. London: Butterworths, 1973.

Northern Peru

Baertl, Juan M.; Morales, Enrique; Verastegui, Gustavo; and Graham, George G. "Diet Supplements for Entire Communities: Growth and Mortality of Infants and Children." *The American Journal of Clinical Nutrition* 23/6 (June 1970): 707-15.

Etimesgut, Turkey

Fisek, Nusret H. "An Integrated Health/Family Planning Program in Etimesgut District, Turkey." *Studies in Family Planning* 5/7 (July 1974): 210-20.
Institute of Community Medicine, Hacettepe University School of Medicine. *An Account of the Activities of the Etimesgut Rural Health District, 1967, 1968, and 1969*. Ankara: Hacettepe Press, 1970.
───────. *An Account of the Activities of the Etimesgut Rural Health District, 1970-74*. Ankara: Ayyildiz Matbaasi, 1975.

Narangwal, India

Kielmann, Arnfried A., and McCord, Colin. "Weight-for-Age as an Index of Risk for Children." *The Lancet* 1086 (June 10, 1978): 1247-50.
McCord, Colin, and Kielmann, Arnfried A. "Home Treatment for Childhood Diarrhea in Punjab Villages." *Journal of Tropical Pediatrics and Environmental Child Health* 23/4 (August 1977): 197-201.
Taylor, Carl E.; Kielmann, Arnfried A.; Parker, Robert L.; Chernichovsky, Dov; DeSweemer, Cecile; Uberoi, Inder S.; Masih, Norah; Kakar, D. N.; Sarma, R. S. S.; and Reinke, William A. "Malnutrition, Infection, Growth, and Development: The Narangwal Experience." Mimeographed.
Taylor, Carl E.; and Singh, R.D. "The Narangwal Population Study: Integrated Health and Family Planning Services." Narangwal, Punjab, India: Rural Health Research Centre, 1975. Mimeographed.

Rural Guatemala II

Habicht, Jean-Pierre; Lechtig, Aaron; Yarbrough, Charles; Delgado, Hernan; and Klein, Robert E. "The Effect of Malnutrition During Pregnancy on Survival of the Newborn." Testimony presented at the Hearings of the U.S. Senate Select Committee on Nutrition and Human Needs, Washington, D.C., June 5, 1973.

Habicht, Jean-Pierre; Lechtig, Aaron; Yarbrough, Charles; and Klein, Robert E. "Maternal Nutrition, Birth Weight, and Infant Mortality." In *Size at Birth,* CIBA Foundation Symposium 27 (New Series). Amsterdam: Elsevier-Excerpta Medica-North Holland, 1975.

Habicht, Jean-Pierre; Yarbrough, Charles; Lechtig, Aaron; and Klein, Robert E. "Relation of Maternal Supplementary Feeding During Pregnancy to Birth Weight and Other Sociobiological Factors." In *Nutrition and Fetal Development,* edited by Myron Winick, pp. 127-45. New York: John Wiley and Sons, 1974.

Lechtig, Aaron; Delgado, Hernan; Martorell, Reynaldo; Richardson, Douglas; Yarbrough, Charles; and Klein, Robert E. "Effect of Maternal Nutrition on Infant Mortality." Mimeographed.

Lechtig, Aaron; Habicht, Jean-Pierre; Delgado, Hernan; Klein, Robert E.; Yarbrough, Charles; and Martorell, Reynaldo. "Effect of Food Supplementation During Pregnancy on Birthweight." *Pediatrics* 56/4 (October 1975): 508-20.

Read, Merrill S.; Habicht, Jean-Pierre; Lechtig, Aaron; and Klein, Robert E. "Maternal Malnutrition, Birth Weight, and Child Development." In *Nutrition, Growth and Development,* edited by C. A. Canosa et al. Modern Problems of Pediatrics, vol. 14. Basel: Karger, 1974.

Working Group on Rural Medical Care. "Delivery of Primary Care by Medical Auxiliaries: Techniques of Use and Analysis of Benefits Achieved in Some Rural Villages in Guatemala." In *Medical Auxiliaries: Proceedings of a Symposium Held During the Twelfth Meeting of the PAHO Advisory Committee on Medical Research, June 25, 1973,* pp. 24-37. Washington: Pan American Health Organization, 1973.

Jamkhed, India

Arole, Mabelle, and Arole, Rajanikant. "A Comprehensive Rural Health Project in Jamkhed (India)." In *Health by the People,* edited by Kenneth W. Newell, pp. 70-90. Geneva: World Health Organization, 1975.

Arole, R. S. "Comprehensive Rural Health Project, Jamkhed." In *Alternative Approaches to Health Care Systems,* edited by C. Gopolan, pp. 95-101. New Delhi: Indian Council of Medical Research. 1978.

Arole, Rajanikant S. "Comprehensive Rural Health Project, Jamkhed, India." *Contact* 10 (August 1972): 1-11.

Hanover, Jamaica

Alderman, Michael H. "Bringing Medicine to the Jamaica Mountains, or—How I Learned One Can't Solve Rural Health Problems from a Planning Room in New York." *Physician's World* (September 1974): 55-59.

Alderman, Michael H.; Hustead, James; Levy, Barry; Searle, Ryan; and Minott, Owen D. "A Young-Child Nutrition Programme in Rural Jamaica." *The Lancet* (May 26, 1973): 1166-69.

Alderman, Michael H.; Wise, Paul H.; Ferguson, Robert P.; Laverde, H. T.; and D'Sonza, Anthony J. "Reduction of Young Child Malnutrition and Mortality in Rural Jamaica." *Tropical Pediatrics and Environmental Child Health* 7/11 (February 1978).

Berman, Peter Alan. "Village Health Workers in Developing Countries: Evidence of Effectiveness and Efficiency." Master's Thesis, Cornell University, 1979.

Marchione, Thomas J. "Health and Nutrition in Self-Reliant National Development: An Evaluation of the Jamaican Community Health Aide Programme." Ph.D. Dissertation, University of Connecticut, 1975.

Kavar, Iran

Department of Community Medicine, Palhavi University School of Medicine. "Kavar Village Health Worker Project: Report Prepared by the Contributing Staff." Second and Final Edition, August 1976. Mimeographed.

Ronaghy, Hossain A., and Solter, Steven. "Is the Chinese 'Barefoot Doctor' Exportable to Rural Iran?" *The Lancet* (June 29, 1974): 1331-33.

Zeighami, Bahram; Zeighami, Elaine; and Ronaghy, Hossain. "Stretching Health Manpower: The Rural Health Auxiliary." *Canadian Journal of Public Health* 68 (September/October 1977): 378-81.

Zeighami, Bahram; Zeighami, Elaine; Ronaghy, Hossain A.; and Russell, Sharon Stanton. "Acceptance of Auxiliary Health Workers in Rural Iran." *Public Health Reports* 92/3 (May/June 1977): 280-84.

About the Authors

Davidson R. Gwatkin is a Senior Fellow at the Overseas Development Council. Prior to joining the ODC, he was with the Ford Foundation, serving as Program Advisor in Population in Lagos, Nigeria (1962-72), and as Assistant Representative and then Program Advisor in Population in New Delhi, India (1972-77). His monograph, "Health and Nutrition in India," has been widely used and has served as the basis for the Ford Foundation's health and nutrition work in this area. He is also the author of several studies on food and population policies in West Africa and India.

Janet R. Wilcox received her Master of Science degree in Nutrition from the Harvard School of Public Health, with a specialization in international nutrition policy. She has also done graduate work at the Massachusetts Institute of Technology and has served as a nutritionist with the Community Health Services in Hartford, Connecticut.

Joe D. Wray joined the Faculty of the Harvard School of Public Health in 1975. He is currently Director of the Office of International Health Programs. In addition, he is a Lecturer in the International Nutrition Program at the Massachusetts Institute of Technology. For seventeen years, Dr. Wray served as a member of the Field Staff in Health and Population of the Rockefeller Foundation, assigned to teach pediatrics and community medicine in Turkey, Colombia, and Thailand. He has been especially concerned with nutritional problems of children and with the delivery of health care, nutrition, and family planning services to low-income populations. He has studied the causes of malnutrition and the interactions of nutrition and infections and family size and health, and has published numerous articles in these and related fields.

Related ODC Publications

Accelerating Population Stabilization Through Social and Economic Progress, by Robert S. McNamara, Development Paper No. 24, 1977, 64 pp., $1.50.

Smaller Families Through Social and Economic Progress, by William Rich, Monograph No. 7, 1973, 74 pp., $2.00.

In the Human Interest: A Strategy to Stabilize World Population, by Lester R. Brown, 1974, 190 pp. W. W. Norton & Company, Inc., for the ODC and the Aspen Institute for Humanistic Studies. Paperback, $2.95.

Population Strategy for a Finite Planet, by Lester R. Brown, Communique No. 25, 1974, 10 pp., $.25.

Measuring the Condition of the World's Poor: The Physical Quality of Life Index, by Morris David Morris, 1979, 190 pp. Pergamon Press for the ODC. Paperback, $5.95.

The PQLI and the DRR: New Tools for Measuring Development Progress, by Morris David Morris and Florizelle B. Liser, Communique No. 1979/4, 6 pp., $.25.

Disparity Reduction Rates in Social Indicators: A Proposal for Measuring and Targeting Progress in Meeting Basic Needs, by James P. Grant, Monograph No. 11, 1978, 88 pp., $3.00.

International Year of the Child: An Incentive for More Effective Development Strategies, by Sarah K. Brandel and Davidson R. Gwatkin, Communique No. 1979/2, 6 pp., $.25.

Third World Women Speak Out: Interviews in Six Countries on Change, Development, and Basic Needs, by Perdita Huston, 1979, 172 pp. Praeger Publishers for the ODC. Paperback, $4.95.

Development As If Women Mattered: An Annotated Bibliography with a Third World Focus, by May Rihani, prepared under the auspices of the Secretariat for Women in Development of the New TransCentury Foundation, Occasional Paper No. 10, 1978, 114 pp., $3.00.

Women and World Development, edited by Irene Tinker and Michèle Bo Bramsen, 1976, 240 pp.; and *Women and World Development: An Annotated Bibliography,* by Mayra Buvinić, 1976, 176 pp. Praeger Publishers for the ODC. The two-volume paperback set is available for $6.00.

Employment, Growth and Basic Needs: A One-World Problem, prepared by the ILO International Labour Office for the 1976 World Employment Conference, 1977, 256 pp. Praeger Publishers for the ODC. Paperback, $3.95.

Growth from Below: A People-Oriented Development Strategy, by James P. Grant, Development Paper No. 16, 1973, 29 pp., $.50. Reprinted from *Foreign Policy.*

A catalog of ODC publications is available on request.
